Allergy & Intolerance

Allergy & Intolerance

A complete guide to environmental medicine

George Lewith
Julian Kenyon
David Dowson

GREEN
PRINT

First published in 1992 by
Green Print
an imprint of the Merlin Press
2 Rendlesham Mews Rendlesham Woodbridge
Suffolk IP12 2SZ

Reprinted 1996

ISBN 1 85425 067 1

Printed in Finland by WSOY

CONTENTS

PART III: Specific diseases associated with allergy and factors underlying multiple allergies

Introduction

Clinical ecology is an American term used to define the study of the food intolerances which do not necessarily fit into standard immunological mechanisms. Some people have used the term environmental medicine to describe more clearly the field in which clinical ecologists work, while others have suggested calling these 'reactions' not allergies, but rather intolerances or sensitivities.

Clinical ecologists are not just interested in food reactions but in all environmental stressors, including reactions to natural substances such as dust, dust mite, moulds and pollens, as well as reactions to man-made fumes and chemicals. Because of their slightly different view of what constitutes a food or chemical 'allergy', clinical ecologists have come in for much unfair and unjust criticism.

Many of the techniques within clinical ecology have been evaluated and examined scientifically, but as with all clinical techniques, some remain difficult to justify on the evidence available. In spite of this, clinical ecologists have repeatedly been attacked by members of the conventional medical profession in a way that seems difficult to understand. While we may not fully comprehend the exact mechanism of a food intolerance, that doesn't mean we can't effectively and safely manipulate people's diet to gain clinical benefit. After all, we don't understand how general anaesthetics work, but that doesn't mean we can't use them.

In this book we shall attempt to give a balanced view of what clinical ecology has to offer. In a sense, clinical ecology is one of the most holistic of the complementary therapies, as it attempts to evaluate the balance between man and his environment, and through manipulating that balance attempts to heal often chronic and intractable problems. Holism means many things to many people, but in essence a holistic approach must allow the doctor to move away from focusing on one specific illness or system and to try and evaluate the illness in the context of its psychological and physiological terrain.

In our practice, we frequently integrate an ecological approach with homoeopathic medicine. Our aim is to identify and treat food and environmental sensitivities, but also to attempt to manage any underlying causes of illness which may be triggering environmental reactions. Sometimes underlying problems are physiological, and on other occasions they may be psychological. The main homoeopathic approach that we use involves homoeopathic complexes. Complexes are not difficult! They are simply mixtures of herbal and homoeopathic medicines directed at either symptoms or specific organs and are the most commonly used type of homoeopathic medication in France and Germany. The majority of homoeopathy used in the United Kingdom involves prescribing homoeopathic single remedies along the lines first described by Hahnemann some 200 years ago. Complex homoeopathy and single homoeopathy involve different approaches and are often prescribed and taken in significantly different ways.

Clinical ecology has been used quite effectively to deal with many conditions such as irritable bowel, migraine, asthma, eczema and arthritis. There are good solid pieces of clinical research which attest to its value in many of these diseases. Ecological disease (that is illness responding to management by environmental medicine) runs across many of our conventional diagnoses. It is very probable that over the next ten or fifteen years, we will find that many conditions have within them a group of patients whose illness is triggered by environmental factors, and can be effectively managed by understanding and manipulating those environmental factors.

George Lewith
Julian Kenyon
David Dowson

Southampton 1992

PART I

The principles of environmental medicine

CHAPTER 1

What is allergy?

Over the last two decades there has been an enormous growth in research and understanding within the fields of immunology and biochemistry. It is therefore important for us to explore what the conventional doctor understands as an allergic phenomenon and to see how this correlates with some of the important concepts in clinical ecology, specifically with respect to food allergy. The science of immunology, the study of the biochemical and physiological mechanisms of allergy, has opened many new doors within medical science and has given us a far more concise understanding of how the body's natural defence mechanism can overcome simple bacterial infection such as acute tonsillitis. This chapter will explore three main areas: our conventional understanding of the immune system, the types of food reaction that may occur within the population, and how these reactions may be explained through the mechanisms that we already understand within physiology and biochemistry.

Self and non-self

One of the major areas studied within immunology is the function or malfunction of the immune system in cancer. All of us regularly produce cancerous cells, but a particular type of white blood cell 'scans' the body and identifies such dangerous instances. The cancerous cells are then destroyed by the body's 'immune surveillance system', and overt cancer develops if this system breaks down. This type of rigorous and highly sophisticated internal health check is part of our natural physiology. Under normal conditions the body is therefore able to identify normal and abnormal tissue with great accuracy; normal tissue is often thought of as 'self' and abnormal tissue as 'non-self'.

Auto-immune disease

Auto-immune disease is one of the areas that conventional medicine has investigated extensively. Many diseases are thought of as auto-immune; this means that the body's immune system is damaging the body itself, resulting in many serious progressive and chronic conditions. In other words the body is unable to distinguish between 'self' and 'non-self'. Certain types of inflammatory arthritis such as rheumatoid arthritis fall within this category, for instance.

Conventional medicine seems to perceive rheumatoid arthritis solely as a disease of joints with an accompanying and excellently documented immunological disturbance within the blood and tissues of individual joints. We are also aware that the disease can have many variable effects on almost all the tissues and organs within the body. Conventional medicine appears to have become bogged down in analysing the disease process, while the clinical ecologist is interested in what event precipitated the disease. Perhaps it might be reasonable to suppose that all the immunological changes that the conventional doctor studies, with enormous investment in technology and with great interest, are purely secondary; by over-emphasizing such potentially irrelevant detail we might miss the cause.

We are not suggesting that just avoiding wheat will 'cure all rheumatoid arthritis'. However, as will be discussed in later chapters, approximately 60% of patients with rheumatoid arthritis will respond to an exacting and careful ecological approach. Consequently we must question the commonly accepted idea of auto-immune disease. All the conventional doctor is really saying is that the disease has an associated immune disturbance. Our experience would suggest that many such immune disturbances are either precipitated or exacerbated by foods and chemicals. Consequently defining a disease as auto-immune has little to do with its cause, but simply tells us about the mechanism in a descriptive and symptomatic manner. It is interesting to consider the observation made repeatedly by clinical ecologists that food or chemical avoidance will often resolve the symptoms from a whole range of auto-immune conditions.

The immune system

The immune system has two main weapons. Initially it produces chemicals directed at the harmful organisms which produce potentially toxic substances within the body. For instance, if a bacteria releases a toxin (an antigen), then the body produces an antitoxin. These antitoxins are called antibodies and are manufactured by a particular type of white blood cell called a B lymphocyte. Antibodies are described chemically as immunoglobulins, which refers to the specific type of protein that makes up the constituent parts of an antibody.

The second weapon is cell-mediated immunity. The white blood cells responsible for cell-mediated immunity are called T lymphocytes. They come in a number of sub-populations, each with its own balance and checks on the activity of the T lymphocytes as a whole. One type of T lymphocyte is called the T helper cell. It is essential for the T helper cell to be activated, so that it may stimulate a B lymphocyte response and thereby the production of specific and appropriate antibodies in adequate quantity. The T suppressor cell prevents the B cell from responding. Both types of T cell can recognize antigens through the chemicals on their surface. Ultimately the balance between helper and suppressor cells controls the immune system and its working in both auto-immune disease and an appropriate immunological response. A further group of white blood cells called phagocytes remove and disperse the detritus caused by an infection. If we suffer from a localized infection such as a boil, pus is produced. Pus results from a combination of the invading bacteria and various types of white blood cell which eat up the debris produced by immobilizing and killing the bacteria with antibodies.

Immunoglobulins

Immunoglobulins fall into four main categories, immunoglobulin E, A, G and M, all of which are proteins and made of a similar basic building block. The major difference between the immunoglobulins is their activity and how this basic building block is bound together.

IgE (immunoglobulin E) is bound to specific cells called mast cells. These are to be found in the skin, lungs and in many other tissues. The mast cells contain a chemical called histamine;

when histamine is released in the skin it causes an itchy red rash rather like nettle rash. If it is released in the lung it may cause muscle contraction, constricting the bronchial tubes and causing a disturbance of normal 'air flow', thereby triggering the primary mechanism of asthma, wheezing. If a specific antigen binds to the free end of immunoglobulin E this activates the end of IgE that is bound to the mast cell, causing the mast cell to explode. Histamine is released and an appropriate allergic reaction takes place.

If, for instance, someone is allergic to house dust mite, then within the lung there will be anti-house dust mite IgEs bound to mast cells. These antibodies will be triggered by the chemicals present within house dust and house dust mite. This means that when the asthmatic breathes in house dust the mast cells will explode, producing histamine, and wheezing will result. This type of allergy is well understood within conventional medicine and there is certainly no debate between conventional allergists and clinical ecologists concerning this reaction.

IgA (immunoglobulin A) is found mainly in the digestive system. It appears to be important in the immune response to digestive infections and may well be particularly important in the mechanisms involved in food allergy within the gastrointestinal tract.

IgG (immunoglobulin G) and IgM (immunoglobulin M) are both antibodies that circulate in the blood. IgM is simply lots of IgG molecules joined together. Both these antibodies respond (with the help of the T cells) to infection with bacterial or viral toxins in the blood, gut and all other organs. Under normal circumstances the T cell system will recognize the bacteria or virus that is invading the body and will trigger the B cell system to produce IgG and IgM. These antibodies in turn will recognize and coat the invading organisms, for instance the surface chemicals on the virus, by binding very exactly and very specifically to the virus. The immune memory is vast and complex, each virus will require a slightly different antibody and furthermore the body will remember any antibody that it has previously made to a virus. Having coated the invading organism with antibody, other groups of white blood cells are then attracted to it; whereupon it is digested by these white blood cells rendering it harmless and non-toxic.

The immune memory held by all B lymphocytes would appear to be almost infinite. This forms the basis for vaccination, as once the immune system has been exposed to any toxin (in however small a dose) it will remember that toxin and be able to respond swiftly and appropriately at a future date. Vaccination appears to prime the immune system to respond to serious infections such as smallpox or yellow fever, so that these infections can be dealt with efficiently if and when they occur, rather than overwhelming the body at their first onslaught.

The immunological mechanism of auto-immune disease involves the body becoming attacked by its own antibodies. They appear to mistake 'self' for 'non-self', thereby activating all the destructive processes normally only invoked by an invading virus or bacteria.

The immune system as a holistic concept

In many ways the immune system is the only true holistic system within the body. Cell-mediated immunity and immunoglobulins are to be found throughout all the body's tissues and structures. If the immune system becomes over-active it can attack itself and cause auto-immune disease in almost any target organ. These diseases are given different names and almost invariably present different symptom patterns, but their underlying pathology is auto-immune. If the immune system ceases to function adequately, the body begins to break down and again many different systems are affected; a good example of this is immune deficiency in Aids-related complex.

The immune system can also be affected by emotional stress. A whole new science called psychoneuro-immunology has developed over the last decade, which demonstrates very clearly that emotional problems change the immune response quite dramatically. For instance, some of the most important prognostic factors for breast cancer are the individual's psychological state, rather than a family history of breast cancer or whether they have taken oral contraceptives. The body of evidence is now overwhelming; emotional states affect the immune system and hence our allergic status. Asthma or eczema may therefore be worsened or even triggered by emotional trauma mediated through the immune system itself.

7

The classification of food reactions

The body may react to food in many different ways, and this has been the cause of much controversy about what does and does not constitute food allergy. Food allergy is probably best defined as an abnormal immunological reaction to food. This means that if individuals are allergic to strawberries, when they eat strawberries an immune response occurs which can be measured in the blood. Such a response is swift, clearly defined and almost invariably reproducible.

Food intolerance on the other hand is a reproducible and unpleasant adverse reaction to a specific food or food ingredient which is not psychologically based. It occurs when a person cannot identify the type of food which they are given, for example when the food may be disguised by flavouring or given as a purée. Food intolerance is not necessarily associated with clearly defined immune reactions in the same way as food allergy, and may fall into a number of categories:

Enzyme defects. For example some individuals simply do not produce the appropriate enzyme to digest milk, and as a consequence always have diarrhoea when given milk. This is due to a deficiency of the enzyme lactase which is irreversible, permanent and often inherited.

Foods that act as drugs. For example large amounts of caffeine have a well-defined insomniac effect on most individuals.

Irritant or toxic effects. For instance irritation to the digestive system may be caused by a curry or other highly spiced foods.

Other food reactions. This is the category that most interests the clinical ecologist. These food intolerances or sensitivities form the practical working basis of most clinical ecology. The immune system does not show obvious changes in response to ingestion of the foods and as a consequence blood tests looking at specific responses to IgG, IgM and IgE are often negative. These tests are called radio allergo sorbent tests (RAST), and will be discussed in more detail in Chapter 6.

Allergy or sensitivity?

Controversies over reactions to food have been inextricably bound up in disputes about terminology. A Viennese paediatrician (Baron Clemens Von Pirquet) first used the term allergy in 1906, to mean 'altered sensitivity'. This basically means any idiosyncratic response to the environment. By 1925, as our knowledge about allergies increased, most of those working in the field of allergy decided to limit the definition, and only reactions in which the immune system was demonstrably altered were classified as allergic. Hence the differentiation between food allergy and food intolerance. Allergy has therefore become a rather narrow science. If a patient does not provide a positive response to a scratch test (a small amount of food is scratched into the skin) or a clear antibody in the blood or intestinal lining to a particular food, then food allergy cannot be the problem to the immunologist's mind. Yet in a large number of instances where no obvious conventional allergy is present, such as coeliac disease, removal of the offending food results in great improvement for the patient.

The clinical ecologist calls this a food allergy as well, often to the sound of derision from professors of immunology. Perhaps food sensitivity or food intolerance would be more sensible terminology, as neither the immunologist nor the clinical ecologist need take offence. We feel that much of the debate that surrounds clinical ecology or food allergy has its roots in the semantics and concepts that surround the word allergy. It seems to mean different things to different people.

The mechanism of food allergy and food intolerance

We have already defined the mechanism of food allergy, and if we accept the narrow definition of food allergy in almost all instances an IgE mediated reaction is occurring, in which the body responds in a known, predictable and immunological manner to a specific food trigger. Food sensitivity is however more complex and until fairly recently there appeared to be a dearth of explanations for its underlying mechanism. However, a number of hypotheses have emerged recently which do appear to hold water and provide some insight into the underlying chemical and physiological mechanisms of food intolerance.

IgE is often found in the wall of the gut and although it is not the predominant cause of food intolerance, it may be involved in mediating the mechanisms of food intolerance For instance, the drug sodium cromoglycate is known to prevent mast cells from releasing histamine. If food intolerant patients take large amounts of sodium chromoglycate orally, this can frequently improve their food intolerance, particularly in the short term.

This suggests that food intolerances may be mediated in some way by the IgE and mast cells in the wall of the gastro-intestinal tract. If activated by IgE mast cells release histamine.

It has been suggested by a number of researchers that the histamine release from the mast cells in the gut wall alters the permeability of the gut to a wide variety of substances, making it more 'leaky'. As a consequence food can be absorbed when it has only been partly digested, so large and unusual food molecules may actually get into the blood stream. These can attract the interest of circulating immunoglobulins; the food molecules are 'non-self' as they do not normally enter the blood stream and as a consequence the immune system will perceive them as an alien invader. Through this mechanism large clumps of protein comprising food molecules and antibodies begin to occur in the patient's blood; these are called circulating immune complexes. These chemicals can themselves trigger a whole variety of inflammatory and auto-immune phenomena through a number of complex immunological mechanisms.

The abnormal food molecules entering the blood stream may also trigger the release of a variety of different hormone-like substances called lymphokines. These chemicals themselves may cause unpleasant symptoms of fever and inflammation, as they are usually only released in acute infection. If however their release is continually triggered by proteins entering the blood through an abnormal pattern of food absorption, then a variety of unpleasant symptoms may result.

Abnormal absorption patterns may also be responsible for the food addiction that commonly occurs in association with food intolerance. Foods to which the patients are intolerant or sensitive are often the ones to which they are addicted. Some researchers have suggested that the abnormal absorption patterns for these foods allow the body to absorb a variety of chemicals which actually give the individual a 'buzz' or feeling of being 'high'. As with many pleasurable sensations, addiction may result as a consequence of over-stimulation, and therefore the abnormal digestion and absorption of food may in itself be responsible for the production of food addiction.

A variety of different enzyme deficiencies may also be responsible for food intolerance. For instance, patients suffering from migraine often have specific enzyme deficiencies. Similarly, hyperactive children appear to produce particular chemicals which indicate that some of the detoxifying enzymes may be deficient in the liver. If this is so then hyperactive children may be exhibiting their behavioural disorders because they are unable to properly detoxify and digest a variety of natural food products. These products may then trigger abnormal psychological reactions through their direct effect on the brain and other parts of the nervous system.

Above all else, however, the body's enzymes detoxify all the poisons which we eat, breathe and otherwise absorb on a daily basis. As our world becomes more toxic, so this enzyme system becomes more stressed. Individuals who have low levels of activity or actual deficiencies of these general detoxifying enzymes (in particular the sulphidoxidation enzymes) seem to be more prone to food sensitivity. The incidence of food intolerance in these individuals appears to be abnormally high, probably because the body simply cannot cope with the toxic load, so any further minor stimulus results in symptoms, one of which may be food intolerance. In other words, a growing body of evidence is emerging that suggests our general level of environmental and food pollution is over-stressing and in some instances overwhelming the body's natural detoxifying mechanisms. If this hypothesis is correct the future must hold an increasing volume of work for the clinical ecologist, as the environment, and therefore the individual, become more polluted and toxic.

Conclusion

The immune system is a complex holistic and finely balanced system. It may be thrown out of balance by a number of stimuli, and certainly mediates a wide range of illness. Some food reactions are purely allergic in the classical sense, however a wide variety of food intolerance would appear to involve the immune system peripherally and in some instances not at all. Food reactions are almost certainly genuinely increasing within the population as the toxic load on our physiology and immunology becomes demonstrably more intense year by year.

CHAPTER 2

Food intolerance

Natural diets

Primitive man lived in a constant and relatively stable environment. Any major changes that did occur were usually the result of natural disasters, such as erupting volcanoes or floods. Initially man probably ate what he could gather, such as berries, nuts, leaves and fruits. As he became more sophisticated he began to develop implements to catch and kill small animals like fish, rodents or birds. Having probably started as a herbivore (a vegetarian) he graduated to become an omnivore (a mixed eater), but most of his diet would still have been vegetarian. Fire, and the ability to cook foods, would definitely have been of enormous advantage to him. The plants and animals that formed the basis of his diet would have been free of chemical contamination, therefore, although the food may have been of poorer quality and more limited in quantity, in an ecological sense it would have been safe.

Poisons

As we have already alluded to in Chapter 1, the increased poisoning and pollution of our environment is undoubtedly stressing our physiology and biochemistry. This in itself will be stressing our natural detoxification systems and ultimately making us more likely to react to foods.

The poisoning of foods, and pollution of our environment in general, began in man's more recent history. Probably one of the earliest and best documented examples is the way the Romans used lead, which they began to mine early in the development of their empire, using it for plumbing systems and in glaze for wine containers. Lead is easy to work, malleable, does not rust and is therefore ideal for plumbing. Until relatively recently lead plumbing systems were a standard part of many large houses, and in some instances they still are! We know from the lead content of the human bones at Roman burial sites that chronic lead poisoning must have been endemic within the population, resulting in symptoms such as intellectual impairment and infertility. Indeed, it has been suggested that chronic lead poisoning was one of the many factors that hastened the fall of the Roman Empire!

More recently tobacco and sugar have been introduced into our society. The effects of smoking are well documented and there are few health problems that have not been attributed to tobacco indulgence in one form or another. Sugar, particularly in its refined form, has only recently received the critical publicity it deserves. It certainly causes serious dental decay and is a significant factor in promoting the overwhelming level of obesity in the Western world. Furthermore, the excessive intake of refined sugar may well be one of the causative factors in diseases such as diabetes, heart attacks and strokes.

Salt (sodium chloride) has been used as a meat preservative for centuries, and in fairly recent history reliable supplies of salt were a much coveted possession. In the past, salt was removed from the meat by soaking before it was cooked, but more recently we have begun to add salt to our food in excessive quantities. We probably all consume three or four times more salt than we need. It would seem that in some instances a high salt intake aggravates diseases of the heart and circulation of the blood; the mechanism for this may be through a direct effect on blood pressure. There is some evidence to suggest that high salt intake causes high blood pressure (hypertension) and that decreasing dietary salt helps to control this problem.

Overall, more than 7,000 individual food items are now in use; many are artificial colourings and chemical additives. Many are mixed into the prepacked and frozen foods that seem to form such a large part of our modern diet. Anyone interested in observing the junk food that is widely available should stand at their local supermarket check-out for an hour or two and watch what people buy. Artificial colourings and preservatives are in regular use to make food look more attractive as well as increase its shelf life.

Chemical and industrial pollution is also very much on the increase. Although in some areas we are improving our environment, other problems such as acid rain are emerging as forceful and destructive influences in Europe's ecology. The use of insecticides, fertilizers and preservatives may be insidiously inflicting enormous environmental chaos, the full extent of which will probably only become apparent long after it is too late.

Can humans cope?

Humans' habitat and habits have evolved slowly and painfully over millions of years. We have been able to adapt to our environment within the context of slow change interspersed with the odd natural or human-made disaster. However, the rate of change has accelerated out of all proportion compared to the past, and as a consequence we feel that the incidence of ecological disease has increased in parallel. Doctors often argue about definition of particular diseases and their incidence. For instance, the nineteenth-century physician did not use the term 'heart attack' as a diagnosis; any chest pain arising from the heart was called angina pectoris. We now differentiate between heart muscle cramp (angina pectoris) and heart muscle damage (heart attack). One could argue that the incidence of heart attacks has really remained constant, and it is just the diagnostic labels that have changed. We feel strongly that such assumptions to not apply to ecological illness. We believe the incidence has increased in real terms and in direct proportion to the extent of environmental pollution both in foods and from industrial chemicals of various types.

Whose illness?

Ecology, naturopathy, allopathy and simple common sense are all giving us the same message. We are polluting our environment and this is resulting in an increased incidence of disease, primarily chronic disease. Man is simply not able to adapt to these environmental changes without some detriment. Not all of us will suffer symptoms; it is just a small but increasing minority which seems to over-react, while the rest of us are able to cope (at least on the surface) quite well. However, it is possible that many of our chronic diseases might be exacerbated by the swift rate of environmental change occurring around us. As a general principle, both the conventional doctor and the clinical ecologist would agree that disease prevention is a better rule to follow than either palliative or curative measures after the disease has become apparent. We would therefore argue that the increasing incidence of ecological disease is one of the many green issues that society has to face over the coming years and decades.

The greening of medicine has not attracted the publicity accorded to many other more obvious environmental issues such as acid rain. Environmental degradation must be affecting the microecology, physiology and biochemistry of the human race much as it affects the macroecology of our environment.

Consequently ecological illness is our responsibility and represents just as much of a political issue as the rain forests, species extinction and the greenhouse effect. The environment that we have all been responsible for creating is making us ill, yet many conventional doctors choose to ignore or underestimate this factor.

If we consider the effects on the individuals, another general principle that emerges from ecology is that the burden of keeping well or being healthy is shifted from the doctor, or the prescribed medication, to the patient. If someone has migraine due to a milk and beef sensitivity, then once the diagnosis has been made the burden of treatment is no longer the doctor's job. The patient must take responsibility for his or her own actions and the consequent symptoms of abuse. This represents a powerful tool within the general framework of demedicalizing illness. Many responsible general practitioners are continually seeking solutions which make patients less 'doctor dependent'. In a large number of instances ecology is an approach that fulfils this need.

However, in spite of the apparently positive and self-reliant attitudes that are an essential part of the ecological management of disease, many patients seem to choose not to take responsibility for their own problems. We could argue the cause of these attitudes at great length, but it is both important and honest to admit that although the moral and ethical principles of ecology in our opinion are excellent, they are certainly not acceptable to all! Perhaps we could say that while conventional treatment of illness is by nature doctor-centred and doctor-led, clinical ecology is by its very nature patient-centred. Treatment in a properly run ecology unit will therefore be patient-led and patient-orientated.

What do symptoms mean?

The patient with food or chemical sensitivity often has multiple complaints. A patient is more likely to go to their family doctor with 'legitimate' symptoms such as abdominal pain or headache; they will rarely consider the fact that they feel lousy and tired all the time as presenting symptoms. Headache is a clearly defined complaint and one that fits the paradigms of conventional diagnosis and treatment. If the patient with headache is asked, then they will often volunteer that they have many other vague symptoms, but do not feel that it is worth bothering the doctor about these. Perhaps they feel (in some cases quite correctly) that many of the other vague symptoms are the product of the severe headaches.

If the initial complaint is vague, such as insomnia, often the doctor's first instinct may be to suggest the problem is a product of anxiety or nervous tension. In some instances this will be the case, but in others, to put it all down to 'nerves' is a mistake.

Within the doctor-patient relationship the doctor starts off with an enormous advantage – the patient is seeking help and in most instances will listen to and accept the doctor's diagnosis and management. If a particular constellation of symptoms such as lethargy and pain are chronic, then almost invariably the sufferer will become depressed and anxious about his continual state of ill health. Consequently, it is easy for the doctor to convince somebody who is unwell that their problems are all due to their state of mind rather than the converse. While an individual's state of mind is of enormous importance, it is sometimes too easy to put symptoms down to anxiety while missing a physical cause for illness.

One of the cardinal rules with patients who have food or chemical sensitivity is that they often present a vague and ill-defined symptomatology. The doctor frequently cannot explain these symptoms as they do not 'fit' into standard diagnostic criteria. Therefore it is simple to convince both himself and the patient that the symptoms signify anxiety due to marital stress or financial worry. In some instances this may indeed be correct, but we have seen far too many people whose problems respond well to an ecological approach to believe a diagnosis of anxiety without looking a little further than the superficial symptomatology.

The ecological history

The classic medical history of a patient with ecological disease usually begins in childhood or in some instances in the womb. Patients who have major food allergy problems from birth often put their mothers through a difficult antenatal period. Immediately after birth, food intolerant children often have difficulty feeding and many suffer with some superficial skin rashes such as cradle cap. At three months they invariably have colic and they then may go on to develop a variety of gastro-intestinal or skin disorders. Upper respiratory tract problems such as catarrh, ear infections, tonsillitis or croup usually occur within the first year or eighteen months and may well become chronic and recurrent. These are often treated with continual doses of antibiotics, which in their turn cause secondary problems such as candidiasis, as we shall see in subsequent chapters.

A period of illness will then ensue for the child between the ages of about 5 and 12. The target organs for this illness may vary; it may simply be the respiratory tract, in which case the child will suffer from upper respiratory problems, chronic tonsillitis or ear infections or perhaps asthma. It may be the skin, in which case eczema will probably be the presenting symptom. Some children become hyperactive and develop a whole range of behavioural disorders, while others may develop epilepsy, both primarily effects on the central nervous system.

There is usually then a quiescent period during the teenage years, or at least a period where obvious illness does not occur, although the child may be moody.

In females 'the pill' or early pregnancy are almost invariably the next trigger for illness. The kind of illnesses that occur here are frequently migraine, irritable bowel and chronic gynaecological problems varying from premenstrual tension to persistent pelvic infections. The symptom list can be endless, but it is usually the biological stress of pregnancy and the immediate post partum period which triggers such further illness.

The general principle we are trying to illustrate is that if people are born with a propensity to develop food intolerance or ecological problems, this inbuilt weakness does not disappear. The target organs for that problem will however change over a lifetime. While the conventional doctor may consider that a child will 'grow out of asthma', it behoves those with an ecological training to ask what the child will grow into next!

The second general principle that can be drawn from these observations is that although the food intolerances one experiences may change a little during a lifetime, there is often a solid core of consistent food intolerance throughout the many illnesses an individual may experience. As suggested, however, while the food intolerances may remain consistent, the target organ and therefore the presenting symptoms may change quite dramatically.

Food intolerances are invariably multiple and often involve one or more of the major foods, which may be disseminated through a large number of other food products. Milk, for instance, is a major food, as it is not only present in its 'pure' form that we buy in a bottle, but also in a whole variety of other products such as biscuits, margarines, sausages, bread and even some breakfast cereals. These major foods often form the basis of a lifetime of problems, presenting a variety of symptoms and having different target organs throughout a lifetime. As patients get older these symptoms tend to become vaguer and more ill-defined, hence the tendency to label them as anxiety or depression rather than seeing the illness as a continuum with an ecological base.

Primary and secondary ecological problems

Patients who have a clear history of ecological disease from childhood almost invariably have a primary ecological problem. This means that they have a genetic predisposition to food intolerance and that such food intolerances start at an early age and usually run in families. Recent studies have been able to define fairly closely the specific part of the gene which may be responsible for the inherited propensity to food intolerance. While the clinical picture in these patients may initially be specific and clear, it usually becomes very much more complex as the illness has a whole series of disparate effects while being managed symptomatically over many decades.

Secondary food sensitivity occurs in patients who have been otherwise symptomless, but may have received some physical or psychological insult which has upset their system very dramatically. As a consequence they fail to cope with their environmental stressors, thereby developing illness which may have an ecological base. The psychological insults which may trigger ecological disease include bereavement, marital breakdown, anxiety states and depression. Common physiological triggers may be serious or chronic infections such as pelvic inflammatory disease, infections of the gastro-intestinal tract such as divirticular abscess, or a grumbling appendix. All these physiological insults may result in a changed immunological response and consequently an immune system that was previously coping may fail to do so. While we cannot explain the underlying mechanism of this, we can observe that this occurs and that an individual's health may be improved dramatically by food avoidance after a period of chronic illness.

People often ask why they develop an ecological problem at 30 or 40, never having had such a problem before. This implies the assumption that one's physiology and biochemistry somehow remain the same throughout life, and will respond in a consistent and totally reproducible manner from birth to death. No-one would expect us to respond to the same psychological situation similarly at 2 months and 70 years old – a combination of experience and vastly different perceptions would make our responses completely different. Similarly, biochemically our response may be very different as we grow older, the immune system invariably changes, as does our capacity to cope with various environmental stresses. As a consequence secondary food allergy can and does develop as our systems fail to cope with the biological and psychological stresses that we place on ourselves.

Masked sensitivity

The symptoms that result from ecological illness do not occur immediately after ingesting the food to which the sufferer is sensitive. As previously mentioned, symptoms are multiple and seem to occur randomly. The ecologist calls this a *masked sensitivity*. In other words, the symptoms are not like a nettle rash or wheezing after ingesting a food to which the patient is allergic; these symptoms occur immediately. In a masked sensitivity a chronic state of ill health develops, such as headache or general malaise. The food to which the patient is sensitive is probably being ingested on many occasions during the day. If the patient is sensitive to milk, then milk in one form or another is perhaps being taken every three or four hours throughout the day. The major problem within clinical ecology is to diagnose the masked sensitivity and subsequently avoid the food.

The principles of environmental medicine

Richard Mackarness (in *Chemical Victims*, Pan Books, 1976) provides a useful analogy for visualizing masked sensitivity. He suggests that the body is rather like a barrel. Usually we can cope with all normal foods and chemicals with which we are in regular contact. These physical stresses can be visualized as water filling the barrel. In other words, most of us are healthy and can cope with most of the stresses (water) to which we are exposed. If we can no longer cope with these environmental stresses the barrel overflows and symptoms result.

This analogy has a number of important implications, which we would like to look at in more detail. Mackarness's original concept of stresses on the body was limited to food and chemicals. In our experience environmental stress is an all-embracing concept and must include much more. A child may have a number of food sensitivities, resulting in the symptom of eczema. For most of the year the eczema may be mild and relatively quiescent, it may flare during the winter (climatic stress) or it might worsen when the child changes schools (emotional stress). Consequently, the events causing the barrel to overflow are multiple and, in our experience, include psychological as well as physical stresses.

Western medicine conceives of the disease as the primary event. The ecologist believes that food or chemical sensitivity is the primary event and the so-called disease (such as eczema) is just the body's response to stress. This idea will be discussed in some detail in a later chapter, but it is important to realize that the symptoms may change while the stresses remain constant. A child with cow's milk sensitivity may start life with abdominal colic and end up with asthma. Although the symptoms may change, the primary cause (milk sensitivity) may remain an important and consistent stressor throughout the child's life.

Another important addition to the simple analogy of water in a barrel is that the 'water' is composed of multiple small stresses. A single symptom such as headache may result from sensitivity to milk, potatoes, tomatoes and eggs. In fact most ecologists recognize that masked sensitivities are almost always multiple and have learned to distrust the observation that 'my headaches are only caused by milk'. In this instance the symptom headache may resolve by excluding milk from the diet, but it may also resolve equally satisfactorily by excluding eggs. The body seems to be able to cope with a considerable degree of stress without breaking down and producing symptoms. The implication of this observation is that not all the foods (or chemicals) to which the patient is sensitive need be avoided. If some of the major stressors can be eliminated the symptoms usually settle and the body will be able to cope with the rest.

The ecologist therefore perceives multiple masked sensitivity as the central aetiological factor in ecologically-based problems. In many instances Western diagnosis is based at a far more symptomatic level, while the ecologist claims to be seeking the causative events for the presenting symptoms.

Hypersensitivity and tolerance

Methods for diagnosing masked sensitivity will be discussed in some detail in later chapters, but if we assume that the diagnosis of masked sensitivity can be made, then a particular pattern of events will follow.

Once the masked sensitivity has been defined the food must be avoided in all its forms. If cow's milk is causing a problem, then cow's milk and cow's milk products must be avoided completely (this would include skimmed milk, cheese, whey, butter, etc.). During the first week the patient will often experience cravings for cow's milk in one form or another, and may even have withdrawal symptoms; these symptoms might include a feeling of tension, light-headedness, excessive sweating, diarrhoea and food cravings. The withdrawal should settle after the first week and the initial symptomatic complaint should begin to improve if enough of the masked foods are avoided.

After the first week, but during the first three to five weeks, ingestion of cow's milk will almost always result in acute and unpleasant symptoms. If the patient's complaint is asthma, which seems to settle after a week of cow's milk avoidance, then further ingestion of milk during this time will almost certainly precipitate a severe asthmatic attack. This is called a *hypersensitivity* reaction and will occur (to a greater or lesser extent) in almost all people with masked sensitivity. This hypersensitive stage usually lasts from one week to one month after food avoidance.

After about eight to ten weeks the patient is able to tolerate exposure to the food. Once *tolerance* has begun it can be used therapeutically in the management of food problems. If the patient exposes himself to the foods too frequently masked sensitivity will develop again. However, if he exposes himself once every five or seven days he will usually be able to tolerate the food and masked sensitivity will not recur. This clinical observation underlies the development of rotation diets and allows patients with multiple or major food sensitivities to eat a relatively normal diet providing they plan it in advance. These diets are called rotation diets and simply involve rotating the foods to which the patient is sensitive.

In a few instances tolerance does not develop and patients may remain highly sensitive to particular foods for many years. In other instances the masked sensitivity seems to disappear over a period of a year or two and the patient may be able to go back to eating wheat or milk with regularity, and without the fear of developing further symptoms due to masked sensitivity.

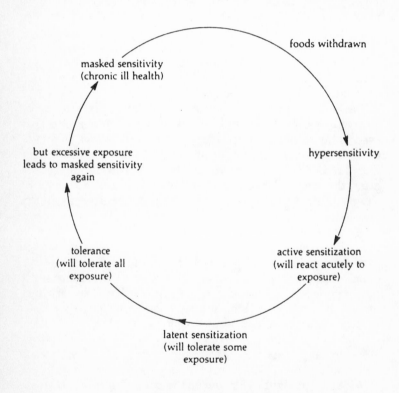

Diagnosis of masked sensitivity.

However, in general, over-indulgence in a food which has previously caused masked sensitivity is likely to produce further chronic symptomatology.

CHAPTER 3

Addiction and adaption

Reactions to foods have been investigated and discussed for the last hundred years. H.G. Wells was one of the first to note the occurrence of food intolerance. He found that if he injected a food antigen such as egg white into a guinea pig, the guinea pig became sensitized to that antigen. A second injection would frequently produce a massive fatal allergic reaction, but if the guinea pig had eaten egg white before the initial injection it did not become sensitized by the injection. It therefore developed oral tolerance and was able to survive the second injection. We now, through our understanding of the immune system, know that oral tolerance occurs, and that our reactions to foods taken by injection are completely different to those ingested.

If you irritate the body regularly but intermittently it responds with a variety of different symptoms. If the irritation stops the symptoms often settle quickly, but should the noxious stimulus continue the body tends to adapt and often only a very few minor symptoms result. Eventually, however, the body's adaptive powers are exhausted and severe chronic symptomatology ensues (chronic disease).

Most ecological poisons, at least from the individual sufferer's point of view, are chronic irritants. Hans Selye has described the three stages (acute, chronic and maladaption) as the 'General Adaption Syndrome' (see Figure). This principle can be applied to all biological systems exposed to a hazardous environment and the consequent need to adapt to that environment. The conceptual models used to explain clinical ecology correspond very closely to Hans Selye's principle of general adaption.

A simple example of the three stages of general adaption is a chronic physical irritant such as a badly fitting shoe. Stage one is a sore foot with a blister; if the shoe is discarded the blister will heal. Stage two of the irritation is the formation of hard skin. If the shoe is worn only during part of the day then no pain or other symptom occurs, but the skin hardens. The hard skin will become sore if the irritation is too forceful, consequently even during the most adaptive stage, symptoms can result from excessive irritation. If the shoe continues to irritate the skin it will break down; stage three is reached as the body fails to adapt.

Alcohol intake often falls into a similar pattern. Most people dislike alcohol initially. Certainly an excessive intake results in the most unpleasant symptoms such as nausea, vomitting, abdominal pain, vertigo and headache. Prolonged excessive alcohol intake seems to have far less effect. Often the chap who has a 'head for drink' seems to be able to take an enormous amount with few obvious symptoms of drunkenness or hangover. This is the beginning of alcohol addiction or chronic alcoholism. In due course the sufferer finds that he can't start the day without a 'snifter'. He feels ill without alcohol and if he goes too long without a drink unpleasant withdrawal symptoms result, such as headache, nausea and tremor. These can only be solved with the aid of more alcohol; the alcoholic is now well into stage three and unless the addiction and consequent withdrawal can be overcome, death will result.

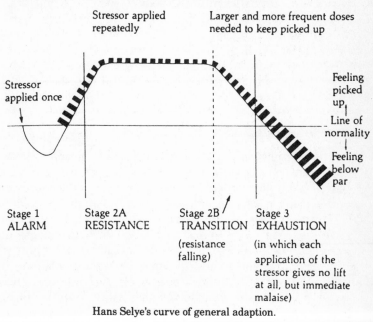

Hans Selye's curve of general adaption.

Addiction and adaption have therefore become intertwined. The body has adapted so completely to the chronic irritant, alcohol, that the individual has become addicted and withdrawal symptoms result if the alcohol is removed. Tobacco addiction is the same; initially everyone hates cigarettes but all too often addiction can result from the chronic abuse of tobacco.

The problems caused by sensitivity to foods or chemicals often follow a similar pattern. A child may find tea distasteful and refuse to drink it, but it may be forced on him and eventually he will begin to like it. The adolescent may become addicted to tea and as an adult may begin to develop symptoms such as headache or arthritis. Removal of the irritant stimulus (tea) may resolve the symptoms.

In many instances, however, a single sensitivity such as to cow's milk will decrease the body's ability to tolerate other irritants. It will 'drag us down', making us less able to adapt to other potential irritants. People usually do not seek medical help until they become ill. When they experience symptoms severe enough to consult a clinical ecologist, they usually have a chronic and unpleasant illness, almost invariably associated with multiple food sensitivities. In other words, single sensitivities seem to compromise the body to such an extent that multiple problems begin to develop as the body finds it increasingly difficult to adapt to its environment. Furthermore the substances to which the body is sensitive often become the source of an addiction; anyone practising clinical ecology will have come across the 'breadaholic', or the 'milkaholic'.

The use of addiction in diagnosis

From the above it is quite clear that foods to which we are addicted are very often the foods to which we are actually sensitive or intolerant. This can be used very simply to help diagnose food sensitivities. One of the initial approaches that can be used to assess the foods to which the individual is sensitive is to ask them to make up a food diary. If they have food intolerance, then the foods which they eat most frequently will be the ones to which they are sensitive. Some practitioners use visualization techniques, and these are particularly useful in children. If you ask a child to visualize a number of common foods, the ones which they feel most positive about and enjoy most are again usually the ones which will be causing the problems. It is almost like the Pavlovian response of the salivating dog, somehow the body becomes addicted to a food which ultimately causes damage, but which is preferred by the patient.

One of the many reasons why the incidence of food sensitivity may now be increasing is because we are able to obtain almost any of the foods we want at almost any time of year. It is only really in the last forty or fifty years that the vast majority of Western people have been able to afford adequate amounts of more or less any food. As a consequence it has been much more possible for us to become food addicted, thereby exposing this inherent weakness within our physiology. Domesticated animals similarly suffer from a less varied diet and as a consequence there have been suggestions by our veterinary colleagues that food intolerance is on the increase. Such problems have not been identified among wild animals, who necessarily eat a much more varied and seasonally-based diet.

The mechanism of addiction

While it is quite clear that there is no definitive answer to the mechanism of food addiction, a number of interesting hypotheses have been developed. Studies published in both veterinary and medical journals demonstrate the initial development of the gastro-intestinal tract is vitally important. Infants born prematurely, particularly if they have a family history of allergy, are far more likely to develop allergic disease if they are not fed on breast milk. A similar story has emerged in the pig; piglets taken away from the sow prior to their proper weaning time, and fed on soya as a substitute, had damaged gastro-intestinal tracts. This resulted in piglets who grew slowly, were more prone to infections and who digested their food less efficiently. Similar experiments have been carried out in laboratory rodents. All these studies demonstrate that in order to get a proper absorption pattern a mammal must be properly weaned in order to allow its gastro-intestinal tract to develop normally.

In most instances however food intolerance does not develop and the oral ingestion of food does not cause problems. H.G. Wells, better known for his early science fiction than his basic science, was probably one of the first to demonstrate this. As mentioned at the beginning of this chapter, he found that if he injected egg white into a guinea pig it became sensitized to that injection and a second injection almost invariably killed the animal. If, however, the guinea pig ate egg white before the first injection, it did not become sensitized and survived the second injection. He therefore developed the concept of oral tolerance which undoubtedly has its basis in the healthy development of the gut and a normal immune system acting within the gut. Any toxin entering the gut is coated with IgA specific for that antigen; this type of IgA is usually called secretory IgA (SIgA). Secretory IgA is then manufactured by B lymphocytes and produced not only in the gut but also in the mammary glands, lung, tear glands and elsewhere. Therefore by exposing the individual to food through their gastro-intestinal tract the body develops an oral tolerance to it.

These two prerequisites are essential for us to handle food normally. The lining of the gut must be allowed to develop normally, and food exposure must involve a competent immune system for us to be able to develop oral tolerance to food protein. If these processes do not occur in a normal manner than the gut may become permeable or leaky to natural food chemicals that would not otherwise be absorbed. The process of addiction almost certainly centres around an abnormal or leaky absorption pattern in the gut.

The incomplete digestion of foods, particularly food protein, may lead to partially digested food products entering the blood stream. These products may in themselves mimic some of the body's own hormones or chemical messengers. One of the hormones which has been particularly implicated in addictive processes has been endorphin, a hormone which has very similar chemical activity to opium. Many food products contain exorphins, proteins that may also have opium-like activity. When the digestion is working normally these products are completely broken down and do not get absorbed and as a consequence do not have a direct effect on the nervous system. If, however, the gut is leaky and working inadequately, they may be absorbed and then can have a direct effect on the brain. The addictive process that is often associated with food intolerance may therefore be based on inappropriate absorption of partly digested food products, which in themselves may become addictive.

Researchers have shown that partially digested wheat can increase the transit time of food in the gut and that this effect can be reversed by an opium antagonist called naloxone, which binds to opium receptors and reverses the effect of opium. Not enough exorphin is produced to result in a full blown opiate addiction syndrome, but enough may be produced to give the food addicted individual a sense of wellbeing. A similar situation may also be occurring in childhood hyperactivity, in that a variety of different artificial unnatural chemicals may be absorbed and ultimately cause a direct effect on the central nervous system. Hence the addictive effect of some foods in hyperactivity and also the bizarre behaviour that some hyperactive children may exhibit.

Conclusion

In susceptible individuals addiction is closely linked to food intolerance. Very often patients will remark that the food you wish to take them off is the one that they can least do without, and this is often a good sign that the diagnosis you have arrived at is correct. There is some good evidence to suggest that the gut's abnormal absorption pattern, which frequently occurs in food intolerant patients, may be at the root of the addiction process. One of the target organs for many of the improperly absorbed molecules is the central nervous system and it is through effects of these products that bizarre behaviour patterns and addiction are almost certainly mediated.

CHAPTER 4

Illness – a revolutionary approach

People often ask clinical ecologists to define the diseases that are ecological, as if food sensitivity always produces set patterns of symptoms which can be described and placed into some sort of pigeon-hole. The honest answer is that many of the diseases described in the medical textbooks can have an ecological basis.

Differentiated disease

The first factor that we have to consider is, 'What is a disease?'. In conventional medicine a disease is probably no more than a collection of symptoms that 'fit' into a classical diagnosis. The medical textbooks talk about 'the classical history of a duodenal ulcer'; this involves central abdominal pain, often waking the patient at night, and worse between meals. The pain is relieved by food and simple indigestion mixtures. In most doctors' minds the diagnosis of such symptoms is a very simple intellectual exercise, but any general practitioner will know that such classical symptomatology rarely occurs. All too often the diagnosis is buried and the story is of vague abdominal pain that is difficult to define and certainly does not immediately suggest the diagnosis of duodenal ulcer. Therefore classical diagnoses, in our experience, are better suited to textbooks than real life.

Does the diagnosis of a duodenal ulcer tell us anything about the disease? It describes an ulcer or a scarred area in the upper part of the digestive tract (the duodenum), but it does not tell us anything about the cause of the ulcer or whether a particular patient is predisposed to the development of an ulcer. It simply describes it.

Common disease patterns

Although the body is a highly complex and ill-understood collection of cells and organ systems, it does seem to have a limited number of ways of reacting to stimuli. Emotional stress often causes us to behave in a particular and predictable manner. It may be that we shout, hide in a corner or go out and get drunk, but for the individual it is often the same predictable behaviour pattern. The cause of the stress can vary from family illness to financial worry, but the individual's reaction often remains the same.

In many ways the body is similar. Arthritis, or painful joints, is an equivalent reaction to that involved in psychological stress. There are two main types of arthritis, active or inflammatory arthritis (rheumatoid arthritis) and chronic degenerative wear-and-tear arthritis (osteo-arthritis). There are a large number of relatively rare small-print arthritic syndromes, but the average doctor encounters such rarities very infrequently. It is possible that many different stimuli can cause osteo-arthritis; the search for the elusive cause, and consequent implied cure, may well equate with King Arthur's search for the Holy Grail. It is probable that arthritic change is one of the body's fixed standard reactions or symptomatic patterns in response to biological stress. For some people with osteo-arthritis it seems to run in families (a hereditary predisposition), some have it because of a broken or damaged bone around a joint and some have it for no very obvious reason. Therefore the diagnosis of osteo-arthritis is no more than a symptom pattern or superficial description of a constellation of symptoms. It is not a disease in the complete sense of the word.

In some instances osteo-arthritis does seem to be helped by the use of a food exclusion or ecological approach. This does not mean that in all cases osteo-arthritis is an ecological disease; but neither does it imply the converse. However, the disease or symptom complex of osteo-arthritis can be alleviated for some patients by appropriate and individually tailored food exclusion. The diagram on page 32 gives a concise summary of these arguments.

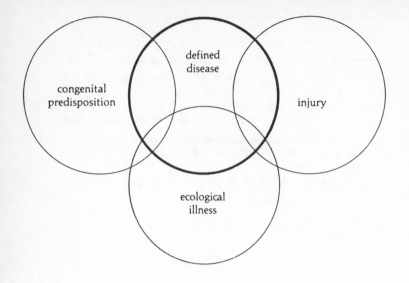

Diagnosis of differentiated disease.

Undifferentiated disease

Undifferentiated disease results in equally difficult problems. If a person develops symptoms that do not 'fit' a conventional diagnosis the difficulties really begin. GPs are frequently confronted with undifferentiated (in the classical sense), and often undiagnosable, conditions. Hospital specialists rarely see such patients, as most GPs refer patients to a specialist only if they already have some sort of provisional diagnosis. For instance, to whom would somebody with flatulence and malaise be referred? Is this a sufficiently serious problem to warrant a specialist opinion? In most instances, however debilitating these symptoms are for an individual patient, the GP does not refer but soldiers on with a variety of symptomatic remedies.

Because the disease does not 'fit', the patient may end up being referred to a psychiatrist. This really represents the doctor's failure as much as the patient's real need. Of course some of us are psychologically disturbed, it is not uncommon. And in a few instances severe distortion of our mental facilities can result in a bizarre collection of symptoms.

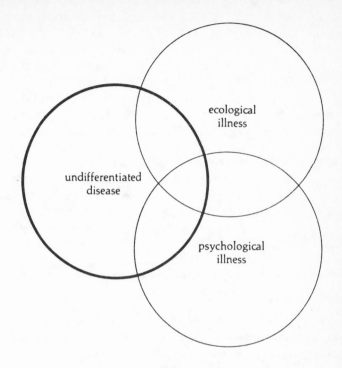

Diagnosis of undifferentiated disease.

Who is to blame?

Imagine the frustration of a trained professional (a doctor) with a problem patient who does not seem to fit into the diagnostic criteria that he learnt at medical school. The doctor's first impulse is not to reject his training, but in a subtle way to blame the patient. He may almost suggest that it is not his (the doctor's) fault that the patient cannot be helped, but that it is the patient's fault for being ill. Such frustration is easy to understand and unfortunately all too common. The patient is classed as difficult, depressed, anxious or mad. The doctor uses his powerful status, within the one-to-one consultation, to create a convincing argument. The end result is that the patient often believes that it really is his fault that he is ill, and 'it's all in the mind'. It takes a strong-minded, perceptive and well-informed patient to authoritatively and effectively contradict the medical diagnosis. Most accept the psychiatric label and develop appropriate behaviour patterns in order to cope.

We are not for a moment suggesting that all undifferentiated disease is ecological, but we are implying that some of it is. Some is clearly due to emotional trauma, inappropriate behaviour patterns or frank delusion. The Venn diagram on p. 33 summarizes this argument. Nevertheless all facets of an undifferentiated illness must be considered and it is perhaps wise to ponder on the idea that it is difficult to consider effectively an opinion that you know nothing about. Without an understanding of basic quantum physics the atom bomb would not have been possible. How can a doctor seriously consider food sensitivity as the cause of a patient's problems if he knows nothing about clinical ecology?

Ecological disease?

Perhaps it would be sensible to reconsider the question, 'What is an ecological disease?'. The answer still remains that many diseases have an ecological element to them. However, the extent and exact nature of food or chemical sensitivity in particular symptom complexes remains an unknown quantity. We have argued that we believe ecological disease is on the increase – not just the diagnosis of ecological problems, but in real terms. It is almost certain that a small but significant group of people are more prone to ecological problems, while the rest of us can adapt to our environment without too much difficulty. We would therefore suggest that an ecological cause should be considered for almost all medical problems and only rejected if such an approach is obviously inept (as in the case of a fractured leg) or incorrect (for that individual patient).

However, the idea that illness can be due totally or in part to the food we eat remains a controversial one within conventional medicine. The reasons for this are not easy to find, as it is common sense that something we do to ourselves three times daily for most of our lives may be a major determining factor of our health. Perhaps two of the reasons may be the resistance to new ideas by modern scientific medicine and its dominant specialist constitution.

New ideas in medicine

The quantum physicist Max Planck said 'An important scientific innovation rarely makes its way by gradually winning over and converting its opponents. What does happen is that its opponents gradually die out and the growing generation is familiarized with the idea from the beginning'. Orthodox medicine is slow to accept new therapies and quite reasonably expects a good body of evidence to be available before these ideas are accepted.

This evidence is gradually accumulating, but unfortunately some of it is conflicting and does not fit in with current theories of disease causation. Additionally, contrary to the textbooks and philosophers of the scientific method, bad ideas are rarely proven wrong in medicine; they are simply forgotten. The true test of a scientific idea is not its intellectual checking mechanisms, but a much more objective judge – time. These factors mitigate against critical acceptance of the ideas of ecology by orthodox medicine, with the result that two opposing camps have developed – the ecologists with evermore entrenched views and orthodox medicine holding similarly entrenched ideas, with neither side being able to look at their own ideas critically.

Specialism

The split into specialist camps is characteristic of the path modern medicine has followed over the past century. There has been, and still is, a strong tendency towards specialization which perhaps explains this polarization. This is probably a reflection of our modern approach to life, in that it is fashionable to be a specialist, and 'down-market' to offer a number of approaches. Unfortunately the trend of specialism has been accelerated by our educational system, with its emphasis on a narrowing of subjects studied from an early age. The 'disease of specialism' has even spread to the patient, who may see a generalist approach, best represented by general practice, as being second class. Specialism does have its positive aspects, but our point is that we feel that it has gone too far in one direction. It has led to vested interest and, in some cases, inappropriate treatment in both orthodox and in some instances complementary medical camps.

The principles of environmental medicine

Vested interest in medicine

The modern trend in cardiology for highly technological and expensive coronary care units is a good example of vested interest. Studies have looked at the efficacy of coronary care units for the intensive care of patients who have recently had heart attacks. The majority of these studies showed that treatment in such units carried no significant therapeutic advantage to home-based care. One study, however, did show a statistically significant difference in results between the home-based group and the group in the coronary care unit; the patients at home did significantly better than those in hospital! These findings were presented (before publication) to the chief of the coronary care unit concerned, but were mistakenly presented the wrong way round (i.e. with the implication that the hospital group did better than those at home). The cardiologist concerned reacted strongly and said that this was the long-awaited vindication of coronary care units. Then the mistake was realized and it was pointed out that the results were the converse. The cardiologist could not be persuaded to change his view of coronary care units.

Specialism encourages a narrow view of illness and engenders a trend to putting diseases into neat diagnostic boxes. The prevailing task of the specialist often appears to be one of semantics, with the initially enthusiastic collusion of the patient in hot pursuit of diagnosis. Once the label has been handed down, often at enormous expense in terms of diagnostic tests, the patient obtains some short-lived satisfaction. When this runs out the true quest for a solution begins.

Ecology breaks all the rules by cutting across the artificial boundaries of specialization and also allows the beginnings of an explanation for the increasing number of diseases that do not fit into neat diagnostic boxes. Perhaps an important feature of clinical ecology is that it encourages a novel and more holistic view of illness, but unfortunately ecology itself has developed into a speciality. Perhaps the disease of specialization is endemic to all medicine.

A causally directed view of illness

Modern medicine, in spite of protestations to the contrary, has a predominantly symptomatic approach to illness. For example, arthritis is usually dealt with by pain-killers and anti-inflammatory drugs. There is little attempt to try to determine and then remedy factors which may have caused the inflammation or wear and tear of the joints in the first place. Ecology offers the possibility of a causally directed approach to illness; in other words, it allows causative environmental factors to be identified and then removed, with consequent resolution of the problem if the diagnosis is correct.

It is curious that there is resistance to this sort of approach within the medical profession. This may have something to do with the constant brainwashing of doctors, particularly general practitioners, by drug companies. As a result approaches concentrating purely on symptom suppression have been given the cloak of academic respectability. The medical management of asthma, for example has been criticized as a euphemism for symptom suppression, often with steroids. To a certain extent this is true, but many asthmatics are also given Intal (sodium cromoglycate), a drug which suppresses allergic reactions. Many doctors would argue that this is a causally directed approach, which to a degree it is. However, if it were possible to identify the factors which caused the allergic reaction in the first place and remove these, then it would be possible to treat the asthma without drugs at all.

A critical view of the ecological approach

The ecological approach to illness has been taken up with some enthusiasm and some lack of criticism by a few doctors and many patients. The result has been that ecologists tend to see all illness in terms of environmental causes. In practice the ecological approach works well for a wide range of disease, but *a few patients* using this approach have noticed some drawbacks, most commonly that the patient, having been better initially, then relapses. The ecologist then assumes that other hitherto latent sensitivities have now come to the surface, and need to be isolated. For a while this approach seems to work as more and more sensitivities are found with consequent increasing limitations on the sort of life the patient can expect to lead. Eventually it becomes apparent that as soon as one sensitivity has been found another develops. The ecologist, however, remains convinced that environmental causes are primary and the patient is locked into a medical (albeit unconventional) merry-go-round.

Perhaps because ecologists have been so beleaguered, they have been unable to ask themselves whether the food and chemical sensitivities are not themselves manifestations of an underlying cause. We shall be discussing a number of such ideas, but remain firmly convinced that the spirit of an ecological approach cannot solely be constrained by the search for ever increasing food allergies or desensitization procedures.

Underlying causes of food and chemical sensitivities

Our work with multiple food and chemical sensitivity has led us to look behind these sensitivities, in order to devise a manageable treatment programme for many of these patients. The few patients who require this approach are those whose problem has responded initially to an ecological approach and who have been successfully desensitized, but unfortunately keep developing new sensitivities. Many such patients, if managed ecologically, lead a more and more limited life and if desensitized may collect enormous numbers of desensitizing solutions, in many cases well over fifty. Because these patients keep developing new sensitivities we think that this indicates we are not dealing with the primary problem but just treating their sensitivities. Thankfully this group of patients is very small in relation to the total who have problems amenable to an ecological approach, but unfortunately it is a growing minority and so it is of increasing urgency that the limitations of an exclusively ecological approach are recognized. However, many of our insights into underlying causes may be provided by these difficult problems.

We will be discussing in the subsequent chapters some of the underlying causes of food sensitivities. While these are not common, they do give us fascinating insights into the interplay between primary and secondary ecological problems. As such, they illustrate some of the basic practicalities of why clinical ecology represents such a radically different approach to illness compared to the assumptions made within conventional medicine.

PART II

The clinical management of allergy

CHAPTER 5

What diseases are caused by allergy?

Allergy causes different conditions in children and adults, and commonly when the same condition is caused, different allergens are responsible. For this reason common allergic diseases in children are discussed separately from those in adults.

Children

A history of allergic disease in the parents will render a child more prone to the development of allergic disease, as will other factors in his/her early life.

Commonly, allergy first shows towards the end of the first six months, with the introduction of solid feeding. Children usually express allergies in response to a particular allergen, rather than being born with pre-existing allergies. As with allergies in adulthood, regular and frequent exposure to an item either in the diet or the environment can lead to sensitization, and the development of a masked allergy. For this reason, if an allergy develops in the first year of life milk sensitivity is probably the most frequent cause, as cow's milk is introduced into the diet on a regular and frequent basis at a very early stage.

Probably the most important factor which may lessen the likelihood of allergy in childhood is breastfeeding. Not only does breastfeeding in the first few months of life minimize contact with foreign proteins which are potentially allergenic, but it also renders some resistance to the development of allergy in the child by increasing the intake of immunoglobulins from the mother. However, it is possible for a child with cow's milk sensitivity to react to breast milk if the mother has a high intake of milk-based foods. For this reason it is probably wise for nursing mothers to restrict their intake of dairy products and make up their protein and mineral intake from non-milk sources.

Apart from the problem of cow's milk allergy due to sensitivity to the protein (usually causing eczema), a sensitivity to lactase, the sugar present in milk, can occur. This normally manifests itself as abdominal pain, or in its most extreme form severe diarrhoea with failure to thrive and gain weight.

CASE HISTORY

At one year old John developed diarrhoea, with unformed stools passed four to five times daily. In addition he obviously had abdominal pain, particularly at night, had a distended abdomen and was not gaining weight.

He was admitted to hospital thought to be suffering from coeliac disease (sensitivity to gluten in cereals), but a biopsy was negative. In view of the fact that his condition was deteriorating, cow's milk was excluded from his diet and within forty-eight hours the diarrhoea had settled. From that time, provided cow's and other animal's milks were avoided, he started gaining weight again, and had normal bowel action.

Specific conditions caused by allergy in children

Behavioural problems

Hyperactivity in childhood is a major problem, as it can cause considerable family disturbance and disharmony. Commonly, at around the age of 2 the child becomes restless, agitated, and has frequent outbursts of irrational and uncontrollable behaviour. There are often temper tantrums triggered by trivial events. Whilst psychological factors must be considered, the possibility of an allergic basis is supported if the child has marked sleep disturbance with restless agitated sleep, and demonstrates signs of remorse after his uncontrollable behaviour. Indeed many children appear to recognize that this is a physical condition, in that they express the opinion that they are unable to help themselves and even sometimes describe it as being 'controlled'. While such symptoms are common to all children, the hyperactive child over-reacts in all environments (home, school and with friends).

Unrecognized as an allergy, the condition develops secondary features which can be harder to treat. An alienation can occur between the child and the parents which compounds the problem, leads to resentment in the child at not being recognized as having a physical condition, and consequent overlying psychological factors in behaviour.

Clues as to the offending item can often be gained from a history of the diet before outbursts of aggressive/hyperactive behaviour. In addition, careful analysis of items in the diet which are perhaps taken to excess may give a clue, as it is frequently ingested items which are often the culprit.

In the 1950s a Dr. Feingold developed a diet for hyperactivity which to a large extent excluded berries and fruit products. This appeared successful in some patients, although the reasons for this were unknown. It is now clear that the Feingold diet reduces the intake of salicylates, and salicylates in the diet are a common cause of hyperactivity/behavioural problems in children.

Salicylate sensitivity is *not* a true allergy. It appears that children can tolerate a certain level of salicylates, but if they exceed this amount their behaviour becomes abnormal. Unfortunately salicylates are present in a large number of foods and total exclusion is impossible as this would lead to dietary deficiencies. Often all that is necessary is to avoid the foods which are high in salicylates. A full list is given on p. 206.

On a low salicylate diet the behaviour of the child can often improve within days. If this happens, attention to any underlying psychological factors must be given, as these may be more difficult to repair. As with other sensitivities, it is usually possible for the diet to become more varied after a few months, though probable that a degree of salicylate sensitivity will remain throughout childhood.

Chronic catarrh
Catarrh is a common problem in children and leads to recurrent upper respiratory tract infections with ear infections and tonsillitis. Usually a toddler develops nasal speech, poor hearing and ear infections. His nose is permanently blocked with

thick mucousy fluid, he becomes lethargic, easily tired and depressed. The energy of such a child is below normal.

Further clues as to an allergic basis of the condition can be the development of 'allergic shiners', dark rings under the eyes caused by congestion of the blood vessels in the upper part of the nose, and the allergic 'salute' – the running of the palm of the hand up over the nose to relieve irritation.

In a toddler the most common cause of chronic catarrh is milk sensitivity, and in these cases typically the condition shows no daily or seasonal variation. However, inhaled sensitivities can be a problem, particularly house dust mite and mould spores. In these cases the condition is worse first thing in the morning, and if mould is implicated exposure due to damp in the house may be a clue. As removal of these agents is impossible, it is only possible to differentiate between the two by testing.

Chronic catarrh can lead to two secondary problems in childhood: recurrent infections and glue ear.

Recurrent tonsillitis and acute ear infections may necessitate the child having courses of antibiotics, and this alone can aggravate the allergy by inducing a dysbiosis (see Chapter 15). Because of this dysbiosis further allergies may develop.

If a child has many attacks of acute ear infection, glue ear may develop. This causes loss of hearing, and is due to the development of thick sticky fluid behind the ear drum. Unfortunately, if glue ear develops allergy-orientated treatment is of no use, as this will only *prevent* rather than cure the condition. Surgical intervention with drainage of the fluid through the ear drum may be necessary. However, subsequent to surgery the identification of allergic causes and their removal or desensitization will prevent a recurrence.

Eczema

Eczema in children often develops in the first two years of life as intensely irritant areas of skin which become inflamed and due to scratching often have small bleeding patches. Frequently so-called infantile eczema, even if untreated, will clear at the age of 5 or thereabouts, but in other children eczema may persist until puberty or beyond. The causes, from an allergic point of view, may be dietary or contact.

The commonest dietary causes of eczema in childhood are milk and milk products, and wheat. This is because these are the foods which tend to be introduced to a greater extent, after breastfeeding, and are usually taken on a daily basis. As has been previously mentioned, sensitivity develops to frequently ingested items. Less commonly other cereals (particularly corn) may cause eczema, as may fruits (especially tomato and citrus fruits). However, probably 60% of dietary causes of eczema are due to milk and a further 30% to wheat.

Apart from dietary causative items, it is possible for contact allergens to cause eczema. The most common of these is probably house dust and house dust mite, with animal products and chemicals being less frequent.

If the cause is dietary then the eczema usually develops with the introduction of items in the diet other than breast milk. If a child is not breastfed, but is fed milk products from an early age, during which time eczema develops, then milk is obviously implicated. However, if a child is given milk products and subsequently develops eczema on the introduction of solids, wheat or the other dietary items mentioned are most likely.

House dust mite sensitivity causing eczema is mainly recognized by the fact that the eczema is worse at night, with intense irritation. Exposure to house dust mite is predominantly from bedding, which is why this is the case.

Some children have eczema due to mould sensitivity. Clues that this may be the problem are in the case history, in that mould sensitivity tends to be worse in the winter months and in wet, damp weather, and that there is often improvement in a hot, dry climate.

If the eczema is due to chemicals, then frequently it is restricted to those areas which are predominantly exposed to that particular chemical. For example, formalin sensitivity will lead to eczema on the clothed area of the body, whereas it will occur to a lesser extent on the face and hands. In these cases chemicals associated with laundry are often implicated, and a change of laundry agents can be beneficial.

Learning disorders

At present there is considerable interest in the causation of dyslexia. Dyslexia results in a child who is basically unable to recognize the written word. Common precursors to this condition are an indecision as to whether the child is left- or right-handed, and muddling of words when writing, especially 'mirror' writing. If not recognized this may lead to long-term learning problems, persisting into the teenage years, and indeed may prove a handicap for life. However, treatment for dyslexia other than dietary is now well accepted and successful.

It seems that there may be predisposing factors towards dyslexia. It has been suggested, and some research supports, that there is an association between ultrasound scans during pregnancy and the development of dyslexia in the child. This is particularly interesting in view of the apparent increase in dyslexia in recent decades, during which time ultrasound scans have become almost routine. It would seem possible that the penetration of sound waves into the uterus may in some unknown way interfere with the development of the brain of the foetus.

Apart from this it seems likely that there may be particular chemicals within foods which might aggravate the condition (see Chapter 9). Of particular interest is the phenolic malvin, and in certain children exclusion of malvin-containing foods from the diet does appear to improve their performance.

Asthma

Asthma is a potentially life-threatening condition in childhood, caused by bronchospasm or tightening of the muscles around the bronchi (the tubes in the lungs). It is a condition which is increasing in prevalence, possibly due to our increasingly polluted environment.

Typically a toddler will develop a cough with a wheeze, usually at night, and often associated with an infection such as a cold beforehand. Although the cold may settle, the wheezing continues, and may result in a distressing cough typically worse in bed.

Whilst dietary factors are sometimes to blame, the most usual implicating factors are inhaled allergens such as chemicals, pollens, mould spores, but especially the house dust mite. If the asthma is due to seasonal agents such as mould spores, this is usually clear from the history, but house dust sensitivity tends to occur throughout the year, though it is normally worse during winter months when ventilation of a house is reduced.

If testing demonstrates that a child is sensitive to house dust mite it is possible to manage the problem in two ways. Either desensitization can be undertaken (see Chapter 10) and/or removal of house dust mite to as great an extent as possible should be considered. To do this, the mattress should be regularly cleaned, deep pile carpets on the floor should be avoided as these harbour house dust mite, the room should be ventilated as much as possible, and dusting should be carried out using a damp duster rather than a dry one. In addition there are various devices on the market both to remove and filter out the house dust mite.

Sprays are available that can be used within the room and within vacuum cleaners, containing an insecticide which kills the house dust mite. These should be used with some caution, as they may contain chemicals which in turn can cause sensitization to the child.

Air filters, consisting of fans behind a fine filter, are also available. However, these have the disadvantages that firstly they are noisy, and secondly the filters are often not fine enough to catch the minute dust particles. A better alternative may well be an air ioniser, which electrically charges the particles of dust and makes them adhere to surfaces. They are silent, economical, and effective. A common mistake is to place an ioniser on a bedside table, since as the ioniser acts as a dust 'magnet' this may only aggravate the problem by attracting dust throughout the room to the region of the child's head. They are best used placed six to eight feet away from the bed.

Enuresis (bed wetting)
A normal child will develop an awareness of bladder fullness and control over the sphincters and muscles of the bladder between the ages of 18 months and 3 years. Although control is often achieved during the daytime initially, night-time control may take longer. If lack of bladder control persists beyond the age of 3, investigation and treatment becomes necessary.

In orthodox medicine it has been demonstrated that anti-depressant drugs used for adults have some effect against bed wetting. The mechanism of their action is unclear, and as they have an effect only so long as they are given, they are perhaps best avoided. A more effective method of treatment in the conventional sense is an alarm, which consists of a pad placed over the mattress which when becoming moist immediately triggers a loud alarm, thus waking the child. Despite the success of these in some cases, some children are not woken by the alarm, although the rest of the household frequently is!

A more unconventional approach is to consider that there are chemicals in foods (see Chapter 9) which are neurotransmitters and high ingestion of these may in some way block bladder awareness control. These are often much the same foods and chemicals as are implicated in other neurological conditions such as epilepsy.

Epilepsy

Epileptic attacks in childhood are caused by overwhelming nervous activity within the brain. In some cases this appears to be caused by a hypersensitivity to neurotransmitter chemicals, so that production of a chemical by one nerve instead of firing off only an adjacent nerve causes activity within a large number of nerve cells. This is multiplied by each nerve cell, resulting in the epileptic fit.

The major neurotransmitter present in the brain is serotonin, and this chemical is also present in certain foods. Avoiding those foods, and desensitization to serotonin, often successfully reduces the frequency and severity of epileptic fits.

Foods containing serotonin are banana, beef, cheese and chocolate.

Malignant disease in childhood

At present it is unclear to what extent environmental factors may be important in malignant disease in childhood. There has been much publicity regarding the apparently increased incidence of childhood leukaemia around nuclear power plants, but this has not been correlated with the background radiation. A recent study appeared to demonstrate that the children of fathers who worked in the nuclear industry were more at risk, while an even more recent study has refuted that fact. It would appear difficult to understand the mechanism if such a connection exists.

It may well be that pesticides and other chemicals which are ubiquitous in our environment these days have a role in the causation of malignant disease. In addition much controversy at the moment centres on the role of electromagnetic fields. Several studies, particularly in America, have shown that children who live in the vicinity of power lines, sub-stations, and electricity generating stations appear to have a higher incidence of leukaemia and similar disorders. It may well be that such diseases near nuclear power plants are not so much due to nuclear radiation as to electromagnetic radiation.

This problem is discussed in detail in Chapter 12, but it is worth mentioning that one particular study, by Savitz in America, showed a significant effect, and extrapolation of this finding would mean that as much as 15% of childhood cancers may be due to magnetic fields from such sources. In view of the fact that this study was carried out in a country where there are restrictions on domestic buildings adjacent to sources of electromagnetic radiation, this figure may be considerably higher in the UK where no such regulations exist.

Whilst the commonest childhood conditions caused by allergy and intolerance have been covered, it is likely that other conditions may be similarly based, but, as yet, the evidence is scanty. Behavioural and learning problems are an area not fully explored, and there is increasing evidence that such desperate problems as autism may be allergically based. It is known that autism occurs from about the second year of life, and that a period of starvation (due, for example, to an infection) can cause a temporary improvement in these children. The basis of this and other 'mental' problems in children may turn out to be simple chemical sensitivity, as yet unidentified.

It is significant that the number of children with allergies is on the increase. This seems to be a genuine increase, and not one which is due to an increased awareness of allergies. This is probably due to the factors mentioned in Chapters 1 and 2, of more widely available foods and increasing chemical pollution. Orthodox medicine has recently recognized that asthma is increasing and that exposure to inhaled chemicals may be the cause. As yet, the increasing occurrence of other diseases which may well be allergically based has not been considered. One has to wonder how long the increase will continue before the cause is recognized by the establishment and national and international legislation is implemented to lessen the pollution threat.

Adults

Whilst the substances which cause allergies and sensitivities in adults are much the same as in children, the relative incidence is different, as are the conditions produced. Clearly the diet of an adult is not the same as a child's in that there are some foods consumed by one group but not the other. In addition the change in lifestyle may have an effect, particularly in terms of occupation, which may expose an adult to chemicals to which he/she was not exposed as a child.

Often an adult seems surprised that a sensitivity has developed when there is no history in earlier life of similar problems. As we have mentioned, problems develop when over-exposure has put a strain on the system. Other factors may contribute to this strain, and this partially explains why the development of allergies/sensitivities happens at particular times.

Stress is an all too common word in our present society. But it is stress, in its widest meaning, that can trigger the development of allergies. By stress we mean not only the daily rush of work and home life, but also the stress placed on the body by infection, hormonal change, and psychological trauma. Hence allergy-based illness commonly starts following an infection (as discussed in Chapter 16), or after emotional problems such as bereavement (see Chapter 17). Hormonal alterations during pregnancy or the menopause are other potential 'trigger' factors for allergies. Although it is highly likely that many other conditions of adult life could be caused by allergy, the most common problems will now be considered.

Specific conditions caused by allergy in adults

Obesity
It seems that true obesity, where a person remains overweight despite a reduced food intake, is a relatively recent phenomenon. Overweight problems due to excessive food intake have long been present. Many doctors find it hard to believe that their patients remain fat despite their protestations that they 'eat next to nothing'. Increasingly, it is becoming clear that it is *what* you eat rather than *how much* which is important.

Frequently a patient will be advised to adhere to a particular exclusion diet, not because of their obesity, but for some other condition. Much to their surprise and delight their weight decreases as a beneficial 'side-effect' of the diet, and often they will comment that other stringent methods to attempt to lose weight had previously been unsuccessful.

As would be expected, the common food sensitivities which cause obesity are those foods which are high in calories. A careful dietary history, with awareness of which foods are 'hidden' in others, may be all that is necessary to identify the offending food, and almost always it is a food which is taken daily. So a patient who has a daily and high intake of bread, or pastries, or pasta together with a liking for wheat-based alcoholic drinks, will probably be wheat sensitive. Another patient who craves, and has to satisfy that craving, for chocolate and sweet foods may well be sugar sensitive.

It seems that in patients with a food sensitivity as a cause of their obesity the particular food may interfere with normal metabolic processes and particularly the action of insulin. Normally insulin is produced in order to keep the blood sugar at a reasonable level, and maintain it at this level for some hours. In the obese person, this production does not occur, allowing blood glucose levels to rise, causing the deposition of fat, followed by a rapid fall leading to a consequent desire for further food.

Apart from wheat and sugar, the other common foods which can cause obesity by sensitivity are corn and dairy products. Both of these may be hidden in other foods (see Chapter 20), and therefore total exclusion becomes difficult. Corn is particularly prevalent in convenience foods, masquerading as corn syrup, vegetable protein, or maize flour.

An exclusion diet for obesity can, initially, be very difficult, in view of cravings for the offending food. But if adhered to for about two weeks the reward in terms of weight loss is often sufficient impetus for continuation.

Psychiatric disorders

The psychological effects of some foods has long been recognized by orthodox doctors, in that an excess intake of caffeine, contained in coffee, tea and chocolate, can lead to agitation, restlessness and insomnia. In addition the effect of alcohol in lessening inhibitions, responsibilities and reflex action is known to all. It is being more recognized now that there are other chemicals within foods which may have a mood altering effect. Unlike alcohol and caffeine, this may be an individual reaction, in that for some people foods have a drug-like effect, possibly due to some error in the way in which they are metabolized so producing drug-like chemicals.

Commonly patients with psychiatric symptoms due to allergy display sudden mood swings, which may be of elation or depression. Apart from foods the most usual culprits are chemicals, especially domestically encountered chemicals which have a rapid effect through inhalation. The mood altering effect of glue-sniffing is well known, but the same chemicals may be encountered at a level at which the patient is unaware of them, but still enough to affect a sensitive individual.

CASE HISTORY

John B. is a successful money broker in London, with considerable work stress and having to travel extensively. He complained of sudden depressive attacks, to the extent of weeping, which, when questioned, occurred indoors, and curiously frequently in taxis. Indeed he mentioned that he could get into a taxi and know he had to immediately get out of the opposite door or he would be affected. Eventually it was found that he was sensitive to the chemical used in air fresheners, which are frequently placed on the back shelf of London taxis. Avoidance together with desensitization succeeded in reducing his reactions. But the main battle was won when he was able to realise that there was a cause for his symptoms and that they were not 'all in his mind', as had been suggested.

Apart from such extreme reactions, more common psychological problems such as anxiety or depression may be based on sensitivity. The stimulant effect of caffeine has been mentioned, but some patients may be so sensitive that even a small ingestion of foods containing caffeine may cause anxiety, or, in extreme cases, panic attacks. Other foods may in certain individuals have a similar effect. Some foods may depress patients, and although the chemicals involved are not as readily identifiable, this reaction is also likely to be due to constituents of foodstuffs having an extreme effect in sensitive patients.

Headaches and migraine

Headaches are clearly a common problem and not always associated with allergy. Other factors which may cause them are stress and tension – both muscular and emotional. Migraines, on the other hand frequently have an allergic basis.

Usually migraine starts at either puberty or around the forties – the menopause in women. There is often a history of migraine in the family, with one parent being affected. The headache of migraine is often one-sided, with nausea, and frequently a 'warning' that it is coming starts with alteration of sensation – usually visual.

It is well known that certain foods, in some sufferers, may trigger a migraine attack – particularly cheese, chocolate and oranges, but sometimes a migraine may occur without these foods being consumed. This may well be because the individual has sensitivities to several foods, which taken separately are no problem, but together on the same day are sufficient to cause an attack.

One of the most common causes of migraine is a chemical known as tyramine. This is a natural chemical occurring in some foods (see Chapter 9) which, even in a non-migraine sufferer, will cause headache if a sufficient dose is ingested as it constricts the blood vessels in the brain. It appears, from research, that there is a genetic deficiency in some migraine sufferers of a particular enzyme which metabolizes tyramine into harmless substances. As a consequence, if enough tyramine containing foods are taken over a relatively short period the level in the blood rises, to a point which is sufficient to cause a migraine. This is exactly analogous to the 'barrel' concept of allergy, but taking it further in that the 'tap' draining the 'barrel' in migraine sufferers is not functioning adequately, leading to a more rapid overflow and production of symptoms.

Nicotine is another chemical which can cause migraine, and it is also present in many of the tyramine containing foods. Often patients with this problem are ex-smokers, who would appear to have become sensitized by their smoking. A clue to the basis of the problem may be found if it has been noticed that headaches occur after being in a smoky atmosphere.

Recurrent infections
As well as infection being a trigger to the development of allergies, allergies predispose to infection. This can therefore lead to a downward vicious spiral of infection – allergy – infection – more allergy, leading to reactions to more and more substances. The overall load on the immune system renders it unable to cope with an infection which a healthy person could readily destroy. Often these infections are due to minor viruses, such as colds and 'flu, so that the patient says that they are 'catching one cold after another'. But more serious infections, such as shingles or glandular fever, may occur. With the latter, long-term illness leading to post viral fatigue syndrome or myalgic encephalomyelitis may result, with further allergies and/or candidiasis developing (see Chapter 14). Unfortunately orthodox practitioners do not recognize the underlying cause of recurrent infection, and tend to treat the infection, if possible, rather than the allergies, so only creating temporary improvement.

Bowel disorders

The irritable bowel syndrome (IBS) is a common problem well known to general practitioners, and because it is not dangerous and does not require hospital treatment it is perhaps dealt with too lightly. However, in some cases the symptoms may affect the life of the patient to an excess level. Typically the patient with IBS has abdominal discomfort, distension and frequent bowel action. There may be urgency in that bowel action can occur with little warning, causing anxiety which only aggravates the condition.

CASE HISTORY

Michael ran his own business selling office equipment throughout the country. This needed a considerable amount of travelling by car. He developed abdominal pain with excess flatulence which was an embarrassment when dealing with clients. His general practitioner advised a high fibre diet, but this only aggravated the wind. Diarrhoea subsequently occurred, often with little warning, and became so severe that Michael avoided driving along busy roads in case he became stuck in a traffic jam and was unable to reach a toilet. This began to effect business, in that travelling took longer, and he began to worry over delays – which in turn affected his bowel frequency. Following testing he was advised to exclude dairy products and not to succumb to his anxiety by avoiding busy routes. With this approach his urgency and diarrhoea cleared, and business improved.

The orthodox treatment for IBS involves the use of antispasmodic medication – to prevent the painful contractions of the bowel – and a high fibre diet. Unfortunately the latter frequently only aggravates the condition, as wheat bran is the usual source of fibre and many patients are wheat sensitive.

In IBS milk or wheat are the most common foods causing the problem, and even without testing it is worthwhile patients excluding these, in turn, for a few weeks, to see if the problem improves. If there is no change, food testing is worthwhile as the majority of patients with IBS respond to correct dietary change.

Inflammatory bowel disorder (IBD) is a more serious condition, and includes colitis, ulcerative colitis, and Crohn's disease.

In these the symptoms are more severe, and there is inflammation of the bowel causing the passing of mucus and/or blood with the stools. Crohn's disease may affect any part of the intestine, not just the colon or large intestine, as is the case with colitis. In severe cases perforation of the bowel can happen, which needs surgery.

These severe problems do not always respond to a dietary approach, but evidence is developing to indicate that they should. In particular some patients have responded to a diet excluding a particular phenolic chemical, phenylisothiocyanate, present naturally in some foods (see Chapter 9). But it needs to be emphasized that this is not the case with all patients, and there may be other, as yet unidentified, chemicals in foods creating the problem.

Arthritis

There are two common kinds of arthritis, osteo-arthritis and rheumatoid arthritis. Osteo-arthritis is usually caused by wear and tear on a specific joint. Persistent damage to a joint or a previous history of a fracture affecting the joint may often predispose to osteo-arthritis. It is much more common in older age groups and tends to affect large weight-bearing joints such as the hip and knee.

Rheumatoid arthritis, on the other hand, is an inflammatory arthritis which tends to initially affect the small non-weight-bearing joints of the fingers and toes. This usually occurs in younger people and symptoms are acute inflammation, morning stiffness and problems associated directly with muscles and circulation. Rheumatoid arthritis may go on to affect some of the larger joints, particularly if it becomes widespread.

There are a number of diets which have been suggested for arthritis. Usually these involve the avoidance of acidic foods, meat and fatty foods, such as milk products. These are general diets and quite often they do benefit arthritis sufferers. However, the essence of clinical ecology is to design a diet specifically for an individual, rather than generally for a disease process. As a consequence, different people respond to the same 'arthritis diets' in different ways. We feel that in both rheumatoid and osteo-arthritis food exclusion has a very important part to play.

A number of clinical trials have been done on the effect of diet on arthritis. Rheumatologists are well aware of the fact that if somebody with acute rheumatoid arthritis fasts for a period of a week or ten days, their joints tend to improve significantly. This occurs in about 90% of patients. Recent studies have been carried out using very limited diets for long periods. These usually involve a diet of just potatoes, carrots and one or two other vegetables, combined with fish and chicken. These studies have shown quite conclusively that restricted or oligo antigenic diets (diets very unlikely to contain foods to which an individual is intolerant) have a statistically significant effect on the progress and development of arthritic conditions.

It is important to note that diets for arthritis often take a long time to demonstrate clear clinical results. Therefore if you wish to try a diet for these common conditions you should persist with the recommended dietary exclusion for at least two months. Both the scientific studies and our clinical observations would suggest that the maximum benefit likely to be obtained from the diet takes three to four months and it is only at the end of this time that you can draw clear conclusions as to how useful a diet may be for your arthritis.

While milk products and red meats may be implicated in osteo-arthritis, it is usual to find that grains such as wheat and oats are more common food intolerances in rheumatoid arthritis.

Gout is a relatively common condition that has known dietary links. It is caused by an excess of uric acid in the blood, which deposits as uric acid crystals in the joint. This can result in an acutely painful joint occurring rapidly and 'out-of-the-blue'. The joint most frequently affected by gout is in the big toe, although any joint may be affected by the deposition of uric acid crystals. It has been well recognized for many years that diets rich in protein are more likely to cause gout, as uric acid is an important protein breakdown product. Starvation causes the breakdown of muscle protein and this may also cause gout. While conventional rheumatologists may question some of the clinical trials relating to osteo- and rheumatoid arthritis, few would doubt the dietary links associated with gouty arthritis.

Osteo- and rheumatoid arthritis are the most common arthritic conditions, but a number of other kinds of arthritis may be triggered by food intolerance and therefore solved by appropriate food exclusions. This includes the arthritis associated with psoriasis. Psoriatic arthritis tends to affect the small joints of the hand and, in many instances, may initially be confused with rheumatoid arthritis. Again, the response to dietary exclusions is slow, and sufferers should persist with the recommended diet for at least three months before abandoning it.

Ankylosing spondylitis affects the spine, initially the lower parts of the spine and in particular the sacro-iliac joints, the lumbar spine and the hip joints. This also is highly likely to respond to dietary exclusion, but again it may take some time before the diet has an effect.

Because dietary exclusion takes some time to act on arthritic problems, aggravations caused by subsequent dietary indiscretion may occur up to seventy-two hours after ingesting the offending food. If you are aware of this, you can link any food reintroduction to your symptoms quite easily. Do not expect food reintroduction to cause an immediate arthritic problem; it may do, but it may equally well result in pain two or three days later. It is probable that the offending food combines with antibodies in the serum, creating a huge immune complex. This in turn probably triggers an inflammatory process in the joint lining (the synovial membrane), which then results in an acutely inflamed joint.

As well as dietary intolerances, there are a number of other important triggers for arthritis. We have noted that rheumatoid arthritis is frequently caused by toxicity. The original offending toxin may be a bacteria, a virus or, in some instances, the leakage of mercury in dental amalgams. If arthritis fails to respond to appropriate dietary exclusions, then toxicity should be considered, as should sensitivity to chemicals and other non-foods.

Hormonal problems

In orthodox terms menopausal and premenstrual symptoms are due to a deficiency of oestrogen and progesterone respectively. Usually these hormones are given as replacement to treat the conditions, but this is often counter-productive in that further reduction of hormone production takes place, by a feedback mechanism.

Oestrogen and progesterone are present in some foods, so intake of these can improve the condition, but these foods only contain small amounts. Our work on desensitization, however, shows that if a patient with apparent deficiencies is desensitized to the hormone she is lacking, this has effects similar to replacement. It seems that in this instance the medication, rather than *de*-sensitizing, actually *re*-sensitizes, making the body more responsive to the hormone which is available.

Foods containing oestrogen are beef, beer, cheese, milk (cow's and goat's), dates, melon, yeast, linseed, soya.

Foods containing progesterone are beef, beer, cheese, milk (cow's and goat's).

Cardiac problems

Heart problems are a relatively small area in the ecological field, but they are nonetheless important as the symptoms may be alarming and distressing. Often they are due not to an allergy, but to excessive intake of foods which have a drug-like effect on the heart. Caffeine – present in tea, coffee and chocolate – has a stimulant effect on the heart, so if taken to excess causes palpitations and a fast heartbeat. Nicotine from cigarette smoke can have a similar effect, and it is also present in some foods (cheese, chocolate, tomato and potato) and likewise can cause such symptoms. Even irregular heartbeat may result, which can be very worrying to the patient, but if transient is not usually dangerous.

Skin conditions

Eczema may start in later life, and clues to the cause can sometimes be found in any alteration in lifestyle, occupation or hobbies shortly before onset. As with children, the cause may be either foods or chemicals – having their effect mainly through direct contact. Occupational contact may be particularly important and a careful history of when the condition started and what aggravates may help in identifying the responsible agent.

CASE HISTORY

At the age of 33, Andrew left his mundane bank job to take over his family printing business. This was situated in a small warehouse on a trading estate, and in order to reduce costs environmental equipment had not been installed. Six months later Andrew developed severe eczema of the face, and sought advice. He, and the practitioner, initially thought that there was some factor concerning the weather involved, as the problem was better on fine days. But testing showed that formalin fumes were the culprit – these are given off by printing ink – and that he improved on fine days

as the main factory doors were then opened. Desensitization
and improved air removal settled the eczema.

Urticaria is another skin reaction which is caused by allergy.
More commonly known as 'hives', this is an immediate reaction,
usually due to shellfish or strawberry allergy. As this reaction
is due to the release of histamine, antihistamines are effective.

Psoriasis is a common skin complaint which is often serious
in the effects it has on the patient in terms of social withdrawal
and isolation in view of the disfigurement. Beyond the fact that
there is a family tendency, the cause is unknown, although it
seems likely that there may be an ecological cause.

Unfortunately, skin conditions take longer to show an improvement with an allergy approach than most other problems.
In a condition such as asthma, the organ, in this case the lung,
is functioning incorrectly but is structurally unaltered. However, skin conditions cause a change in the skin structure and
the skin has to heal from within. Improvement may therefore
take months and demand considerable perseverance from the
individual, particularly if his diet is difficult.

Neurological problems
As there is an increasing incidence of motor neurone disease,
multiple sclerosis and Alzheimer's disease these may turn out
to be environmentally caused. However, it looks as if they may
be due directly to toxicity (see Chapter 13) rather than to an
idiosyncratic reaction by specific individuals.

Miscellaneous conditions
There are a number of other medical conditions which are
difficult to treat conventionally but which can respond to an
ecological approach. Amongst these are tinnitus, a persistent
buzzing in the ears, which frequently fails to respond to
orthodox medicine and can be very distressing. Chronic sin-
usitis is often treated by surgery, but this can be avoided if the
environmental factors involved can be identified – commonly a
mould and yeast sensitivity.

Undifferentiated disease
The concept of undifferentiated disease is not recognized by
orthodox medicine, as has been fully discussed in Chapter 4.
Patients may show a variety of symptoms, often affecting

different systems of the body, which appear unconnected. Due to increased specialization in medicine, they may be referred to different specialists for each problem. So they may see a rheumatologist for joint pain, a physician for abdominal bloating, and a dermatologist for a rash.

Each specialist will only deal with one problem, blind to the fact that all the symptoms could be due to the same underlying condition. In this way the patient ends up being treated in a *symptomatic* way for his complaint, and none of the many doctors he/she sees is able to consider that the symptoms may have a common cause. As it is hoped we have shown, it is only with a totally holistic approach that such problems can be successfully tackled.

Clinical research

Within clinical ecology there are two main areas of research. Firstly the basic mechanisms, which have been outlined in some detail in Chapter 1, and secondly clinical research, the implications of which have been discussed in each section pertaining to specific diseases. Attempting to understand the basic mechanisms of clinical ecology, and how environmental stressors may affect the biochemistry, physiology and immune system within the body, can be achieved almost exclusively by the use of well validated conventional scientific techniques. However, within the area of clinical research new study methods need to be adopted as a double blind drug trial is not amenable to a direct transplant into the area of clinical ecology.

The golden rules of clinical trials
Within the assumptions of clinical ecology there are fundamentally two golden rules which must be adhered to whenever one is attempting to prove beyond a shadow of a doubt that food intolerance is responsible for a specific illness. The first is that symptoms should clear with specific food avoidance. If all assumptions about clinical ecology are correct then food abstinence for between six to eight weeks should produce a sustained and clear improvement in the patient's symptomatology. Secondly, food reintroduction over a period of two weeks should then trigger the reappearance of all the previous symptoms. This seems very simple, but in fact it is very difficult to prove.

The first problem devolves around the very nature of clinical ecology itself. If for instance somebody is an asthmatic who is affected by five common foodstuffs, then we can demonstrate an improvement in the asthma by removal of these foodstuffs from the diet. If however the patient also has added sensitivities which are seasonably variable, for instance sensitivity to grass pollens or mould spores, then the problem can become much more complicated. This means that we can only run our food study during the specific times in which these inhaled items are not present and therefore will not confuse the issue by worsening the asthma while we are trying to control it with a diet. Patients suffering from ecological problems are almost always complex and basing all our research methodology on fairly simplistic assumptions such as those that can be easily made for food sensitivity, may be both misplaced and misleading.

A control group

In almost all proper scientific studies a control group is needed. In this group the patients are given an ineffective treatment and then compared with a group of patients receiving an effective treatment. Consequently the investigator can assess in equal groups (as far as that can be achieved) the natural history of the illness and the likely placebo response. The placebo response is probably best defined as an improvement in the illness being studied because of the fact that it is being studied.

Control groups within clinical ecology are very difficult to achieve. We can either pretend to give somebody a diet that is relevant for their condition or use our control groups in food reintroduction. If we put all the patients with a given condition on a diet specific for them, having used some method of food testing based on individual response, we should be able to get a significant improvement in a group of patients with a uniform condition such as eczema. We could then introduce some of the group to foods we know are likely to make them worse and leave the others on their diets to see if they improve. In this way, by rechallenging patients in a controlled manner, we should be able to achieve a valid scientific comparison of two groups and thereby evaluate the efficacy of our treatment.

However, life isn't always that simple. How do we reintroduce the foods without the patient's knowing? We can use food capsules stuffed with the offending food to which the patient may be allergic, but there are a number of problems associated with this. For instance the food is only released quite far on in the gastro-intestinal tract as the capsules need to be digested. Some ecologists suggest this is not scientifically valid in order to get a food reaction absorption from the mouth and certainly the stomach is an important part of the process. Furthermore, it is very difficult to manufacture capsules which do not have some taste associated with them, and as a consequence the patient may know whether they are receiving a safe or unsafe food. We can mask foods by making very complex soups and then putting into those soups quantities of food to which the patient may react. Again masking is complex and difficult and sometimes technically impossible to achieve with the full range of foods one would wish to investigate.

The problem of a control group are therefore enormous and very few properly controlled studies have ever been achieved within the field of clinical ecology. As a consequence most of the evidence that we have to go on, and which forms the basis of our ideas in terms of evaluating if specific illness may be affected by food intolerance, is based on descriptive studies.

Descriptive studies

Descriptive studies are probably the least effective way to investigate illness scientifically. This simply involves taking a large number of patients with a specified illness such as arthritis or asthma and then putting them on specific food exclusions. In most instances the studies that have been published in this area of clinical ecology have put patients on very simple caveman diets rather than attempting to evaluate each individual's specific food sensitivities.

Patients will tend to be placed on a diet that involves lamb, pears, carrots, brown rice and perhaps one or two other vegetables. This works for most patients, but everybody knows what is going on, so no control group is involved and both the patient and doctor are completely aware of the treatment being given. From all the information we have about placebo response, this tends to maximize the placebo effect and therefore inevitably produces a far better result than one would have expected in a properly controlled study, when neither the patient nor the doctor was aware as to whether they were receiving effective or ineffective treatment (this is usually called a double blind study because patients and doctors are both blind to treatment).

Non-food sensitivities

The investigation of non-food sensitivities is in many ways even more complex than that of food sensitivities. First we need to use often unconventional methods to diagnose non-food sensitivities and then superimposed on that we use a homoeopathic or minimal dose therapy to desensitize patients (the Miller technique). Two assumptions are therefore being made which are often unacceptable to the conventional scientific community. Firstly the method of investigation and diagnosis of the specific end point is open to many questions, and secondly the medication used is thought by a number of conventional doctors to be totally ineffective and based on invalid pharmacological assumptions. As a consequence the clinical investigation of inhaled or contact sensitivities starts off with more inherent difficulties than that of food sensitivities.

However, it is far easier to investigate non-food sensitivities in the context of a double blind controlled trial. Since you are giving the patient medication, you can follow almost exactly the same protocol as that used by pharmacologists studying conventional medication. The few studies that have been achieved using this methodology suggest that the Miller technique desensitization (Chapter 10) is both a useful and valid approach to desensitization.

Conclusion

While at first it may seem fairly simple to investigate food intolerance using clinical trials, the vast majority of the investigative studies published have involved soft data and have been based on descriptive studies. These publications have to date not convinced the conventional medical community that we are dealing with valid phenomena. However, the disease we are studying is complex and difficult and the research methods available to us, along with the criterion set for a high degree of scientific validity, are complex. Furthermore little research money has been pumped into clinical ecology in order to develop new techniques of investigation. As a consequence, while much research is available within this field, only a small proportion of it is of a high scientific standard and far more effort needs to be applied to the clinical investigation as well as the basic scientific research if we are to understand and use ecological techniques on a more widespread basis.

The clinical management of allergy

We have introduced many conditions which can be caused by allergy/intolerance and given some insight into the problems surrounding the investigation of patients with allergic conditions. Although environmental medicine is in its infancy the potential, both in terms of problems which can be helped, and further research is considerable.

CHAPTER 6

The diagnosis of food sensitivities

The first question to answer in any problem which is thought to be wholly or partially due to food and/or chemical sensitivities is whether there is any improvement on avoiding appropriate foods and/or chemicals (see Chapter 3). From a practical point of view there is a vast array of foods and chemicals which could cause any problem, and so what is needed is some sort of testing technique in order to decide which foods or chemicals to avoid. In the case of chemicals, complete avoidance is often not possible, for instance if somebody is reacting to petrol and diesel fumes, in which case desensitization is important.

A number of testing techniques are available, some conventional, some unconventional. Unfortunately, the conventional testing techniques are largely noted for their inability to be clinically useful. They are good at picking out sensitivities to airborne allergens such as from cats and dogs, pollens, feathers, etc., but not at picking out food sensitivities. Many trials carried out by the American clinical ecologists have found this to be the case.

The unconventional testing techniques are by far the most successful, and it is very likely that if you do consult a practitioner who looks at food and chemical sensitivity, you will be tested with one or a number of the techniques mentioned in this chapter. Unconventional techniques are about 70% accurate, as a recent paper from Canada showed, but they are highly controversial, and very difficult indeed to prove. Such research as there is into these methods of testing is consistently positive, but we feel that very much more research needs to be done into these testing techniques. Their basic mechanism of action appears to involve a subtle change in the electromagnetic field surrounding the body, which is then sensed by the body and is picked up by weakening the muscle, an electrical response over an acupuncture point or a change in the pulse. None of these concepts are accepted or even remotely considered by conventional medical science, therefore all these techniques are put in the scientific dustbin by conventional medical scientists. The fact remains that they do work and they are clinically useful.

It is our belief that it is only a matter of time before the mechanisms underlying these techniques are more fully understood by medical science and thus they will be more accepted. It is relevant to note in this context that we still do not know how general anaesthesia works, we simply accept it, we use it all the time and we know that it does work.

Conventional testing methods

Skin prick tests
This is the most commonly used test for allergy and looks at how the skin reacts to a tiny amount of a suspected substance. An extract of the substance is used, having been prepared from a pure sample of a food, a pollen, a mould or animal hair. A drop of this extract is placed on the arm and a prick or scratch is made in the skin below the drop. A minute amount of the suspected substance enters the skin and if the patient is sensitive to it, there will be a marked reaction known as a wheal and flair response. This testing method is an accurate indicator of allergy to airborne substances such as pollens, dust and fungal spores. It is not good at diagnosing allergy and/or sensitivity to foods or chemicals. Various authorities rate the diagnostic success of conventional skin prick tests as described for foods or chemicals as ranging from 18-40%, hardly good enough to establish an accurate diagnosis.

RAST
RAST stands for radio allergo sorbent test and is a method of locating specific antibodies to foods in the blood serum; in other words, it defines true allergic reactions to foods. A leading article in the British Medical Journal (April, 1983) on food allergy cast doubt on the diagnostic value of RAST testing for food sensitivity; indeed, specific antibodies to common foods are often found in the serum of apparently non-food allergic patients. There is little correlation between positive RAST tests followed by subsequent food avoidance of the implicated foods

and clinical improvement of the patient. This interesting finding casts doubt on food sensitivity having an immunological basis. One of the drawbacks of RAST, quite apart from its clinical irrelevance, is that the tests are expensive. Some doctors doggedly stick to RAST testing and are reluctant to admit to a sensitivity occurring outside this testing procedure. This has to be a narrow-minded approach, and it is certainly bad news for the frustrated patient who might find himself relegated to the psychological dustbin.

Unconventional testing techniques

Provocative intradermal testing
If the allergens are diluted with salt water in steps of five (i.e. dilution number one is diluted five times, dilution number two is diluted twenty-five times and so on) and these dilutions are injected just underneath the skin, reactions begin to appear. This same method can be used simply putting drops under the tongue, called sublingual testing. Often the patient develops symptoms related to their complaint, such as headache or abdominal pain, at the same time.

For example, a patient may produce no positive whealing response to the injection of a wheat concentrate, but if this is diluted in steps of five, then one of the dilutions – often the first – will produce a positive whealing response if the patient is sensitive to wheat. Within the framework of conventional allergy, this phenomenon is inexplicable – no whealing on injection of a concentrate but a positive whealing response on injection of a dilution. Yet it is repeatedly observed and has been used by us in the past as a diagnostic technique with identical findings.

The majority of patients (about 70%) develop symptoms together with a positive whealing response. Increasing dilutions are usually injected at approximately ten minute intervals until the dilution which produces no whealing (the so-called first negative wheal) is reached. This is often accompanied by an almost instantaneous 'switch-off' of symptoms. This dilution can then be used as a 'switch-off' drop, to enable the patient to eat small amounts of the offending food or come into contact with the offending chemical after having first taken an appropriate 'switch-off' drop under the tongue.

We have no explanation as to why a dilution of a substance can switch-off a patient's reaction to that substance and this observation must join the host of unexplained observations made by people working in the area of food and chemical sensitivity. The fact that the technique works at all remains something of an enigma to many people working with it. This technique has become known as the Miller technique, after an American doctor, Dr. Joe Miller, who first devised it in the early 1960s.

The Miller technique therefore provides a diagnostic and therapeutic approach to food and chemical sensitivity rolled into one, and is the mainstay of many food and chemical sensitivity clinics, but unfortunately it has many disadvantages. It is very time-consuming and often encourages an unhealthy introspection on the part of the patient to his problem. It is also very expensive indeed, due to the many substances which need to be tested and the time that this takes. Desensitization using this technique tends to be very specific, in other words it generally is not possible to give one 'switch-off' drop for a group of related substances, so many substances need to be tested. Also, some patients find that they continually develop new sensitivities. It is therefore a useful yet unwieldly diagnostic technique, and probably is a less than perfect method for treating and diagnosing food and chemical sensitivity.

This method, however, has generated an enormous amount of controversy and acrimony between conventional medicine and those practising food and chemical sensitivity. Such debate is reflected in the recent decision of the health care administration in America to discontinue medicare reimbursement for the Miller technique, which in America is now known as provocation-neutralization therapy. This in spite of the fact that there are eleven published double blind studies, and one animal study, confirming the effectiveness of this method. This action is one of the many clear statements of prejudice against this developing area of medicine, and it is particularly disappointing to find that a properly argued academic case based upon well conducted clinical studies is not a sufficient basis for this method to be accepted.

Cytotoxic testing

In this test, live white blood cells are exposed to a range of foods and chemicals. The presence or absence and degree of damage caused to these cells is an indicator of the presence of food and/ or chemical sensitivity and gives some indication as to its degree. For example, if the white cells only increase in size and become rounded (they normally have an irregular shape) then this indicates a mild reaction. If the white cells burst, this indicates a severe reaction.

One of the many limitations of this test is that the presence and degree of white cell damage is a matter of opinion on the part of the laboratory technician and results can be difficult to interpret. The main disadvantages are that it often reveals too many sensitivities, usually more than thirty, and it is expensive, often costing more than £150 for a reasonable spread of foods.

The correlation between food and/or chemical avoidance and clinical improvement is high for cytotoxic testing; this test is said to be approximately 70% accurate. Some recent laboratory evidence has lent support to testing methods such as this. Cytotoxic testing is really on the borderline between conventional and unconventional testing. We feel that this test may ultimately become more sophisticated, and may be the first effective clinically accepted method of food and chemical sensitivity testing.

Coca pulse test

This is a very simple pulse test discovered by Dr. Coca, an American doctor, working some thirty years ago. He found that the pulse rate increases by ten or more beats per minute following ingestion of an allergic or a sensitive food or exposure to a chemical to which the patient is sensitive. It is a very simple method which anybody can use following fasting and then reintroduction of foods (see page 73).

Clinical testing using the auricular cardiac reflex (ACR)

The ACR is a physical sign used in the branch of ear acupuncture known as auricular medicine, hence its odd sounding name. First noticed by Dr. Paul Nogier, it is a small movement of the position where the wrist pulse is strongest, either in the direction of the elbow (a so-called negative ACR) or in the direction of the wrist (a so-called positive ACR). The ACR changes in response to small changes in the body's energy field. This has been adapted to food and chemical sensitivity testing, and it has been noted that when bringing a dried food or a bottle with a chemical to which the patient is sensitive near to the body (within half an inch of the skin but not touching) the ACR will change.

It is hard to believe that bringing a substance near to the body, but without touching it, can cause a subtle change in the patient. Some scientific backing for this technique comes from studying subtle electromagnetic change around the body and from recent theoretical and experimental work showing that the body is very sensitive to radiation in the millimetre/centimetre waveband of the electromagnetic spectrum.

In experienced hands the ACR test is approximately 70% accurate. Its advantages are that it is quick (fifty foods or chemicals can be tested within fifteen minutes), it only requires dried food samples or bottles with chemicals in, and it is cheap. Its disadvantages are that it requires some training in order to be able to detect accurately, and there are some doctors who find it impossible to pick up the clinical signs of the change of pulse, in the same way that some doctors find heart murmurs almost impossible to hear.

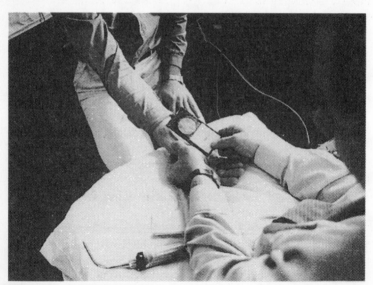

Clinical testing using the ACR.

Muscle testing (applied kinesiology)

This method assesses the changes in muscle strength with hand contact, or under the tongue contact, of the suspected foods or chemicals. The food or chemical to be tested is placed in the hand or under the tongue of the subject. A muscle is chosen to assess any alteration in power due to the patient's contact with the test substance. The food or chemical to which the subject is sensitive will weaken muscle power, and those which the patient needs will strengthen it. Like the ACR method it produces reliable and clinically useful results in experienced hands.

A simple modification of muscle testing is the sphygomanometer test. This can be done using a blood pressure testing machine which has a mercury column. Blow up the cuff which normally goes around the arm and then tie it in a knot, to form a small ball which can be placed in the palm of the hand. Squeeze this as hard as possible and notice how far up you can push the mercury. Then one by one put the suspected foods or chemicals underneath the tongue. Those to which you are sensitive will reduce the height to which you can push the mercury.

This is a very useful and simple test, and is often effective in fairly unskilled hands. It can be carried out at home and is very useful for children.

Electrical testing for food and chemical sensitivity (Vegatesting)

The rapid 'switch-off' of symptoms, found when determining neutralizing drops in the Miller technique, has been observed by many doctors who have used this method. It has been surmised that the switch-off is too rapid for it to have been mediated by a biochemical change in the body, and that an electrical mechanism of some sort is more likely. Not surprisingly, therefore, electrical testing for food and chemical sensitivity is a practical possibility. These methods owe their origin to electrical measurement techniques over acupuncture points and the observation that these measurements vary if a substance relevant to the patient is placed, inside a glass container, in series in the circuit.

This interesting phenomenon is difficult to explain using classical electromagnetic theory, yet it remains a useful method for testing either for therapy or diagnosis.

The clinical management of allergy

A normal reading is obtained over a specific acupuncture point, then a control substance in a glass bottle is introduced into the circuit, which should always lower the reading on the subsequent measurement of the point. The control substance used is usually a poison of some sort, i.e. something that will harm the body if taken internally. Then each food or chemical is placed one by one on the testing plate, which is live and in series with the circuit. Those that lower the reading are the ones to which the patient is sensitive. Those that do not lower the reading are safe. The method can also be used to determine desensitization end points.

The advantages of this method are that it is quick, cheap to perform, and carries a certain placebo effect in that the patient can see the reading change on the meter when foods or chemicals to which he/she is sensitive are in circuit. Patients have confidence in this method, probably because of this, and they are therefore more likely to follow a rigorous avoidance of the relevant foods or chemicals than when using other diagnostic methods.

Its disadvantages are that the equipment (a Vegatest device) required is expensive, although it represents a once-only purchase. Also the technique requires considerable skill in order to carry it out effectively. Like the ACR method and indeed

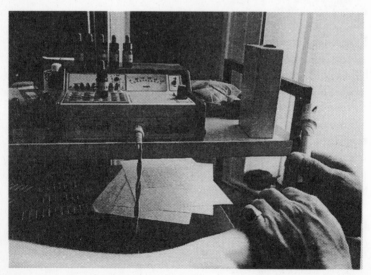

Electrical testing using the Vegatest.

muscle testing, a small proportion of doctors are unable to use it effectively. In skilled hands it is approximately 70% accurate like all the other unconventional methods discussed.

The mechanism of action for the Vegatest method is probably a subtle electromagnetic interaction of the patient's field, the practitioner's field and the field emitted by the substance placed in circuit. It is very likely that this effect is frequency dependent, i.e. dependent on a particular frequency range within the electromagnetic spectrum and this is most likely to be the millimetre/centimetre wave range of the electromagnetic spectrum. When a patient is sensitive to a substance being tested, these fields interact and the reading is lowered.

Elimination dieting

This is a long-standing and probably the most commonly used method of diagnosing food sensitivity. The patient is asked to fast and drink spring water only for five days. Some practitioners allow the patient to eat foods which are rarely implicated in illness due to foods, such as lamb, pears or kiwi fruit, etc. In our opinion a five day spring water fast is the most effective method. It is interesting to note that similar fasting rituals form integral parts of some ancient systems of medicine such as Ayurvedic medicine. The implication of fasting in these systems of medicine is that it cleanses the body of toxins.

If symptoms are improved or disappear towards the end of the five day fast, it can be assumed that the patient's illness is due to one or a number of foods which he or she was eating. Symptoms often worsen on days 2, 3 or 4 of the fast, a phenomenon reminiscent of a withdrawal reaction so commonly found when people try to stop smoking or when an alcoholic stops drinking. The majority of books about food sensitivity stick to the five day elimination diet as being the method of choice. In our view it has a number of limitations, the main one being that not all the symptoms will clear up after a five day fast and a much longer period of avoidance may be necessary, particularly in diseases such as rheumatoid arthritis. If a patient's symptoms are wholly or partially due to chemical exposure, then food elimination will often reveal nothing of any clinical use.

Following the five day fast, the patient is told to reintroduce the foods he or she was previously eating, one at a time. The less commonly eaten foods should be reintroduced first and each meal should consist of only one food, such as eggs, fish, oranges, wheat, etc. If symptoms recur after a meal, the food which is added at that meal is clearly implicated. This procedure is continued until all the foods have been reintroduced one by one, so that a list of food sensitivities is built up; it is important to remember that tap water should be considered for testing as well. It is usually adequate to reintroduce each food meal by meal rather than on a daily basis, as following the five day fast the patient will be in a hypersensitive state and therefore more likely to produce a rapid and definite reaction. If there is a reaction then clearly the patient should consider that he/she is hypersensitive to this food and exclude it from their diet.

This method breaks down in those patients who react twenty-four hours after taking a food to which they are sensitive. The most delayed reaction we have ever encountered is one of forty-eight hours. Clearly, using an elimination dieting technique in these delayed reactors is a cumbersome and time-consuming procedure. The technique is difficult enough to manage even in those who do react quickly on reintroduction of foods.

The major drawback of this method, in our view, is that results are often confusing, and certainly not as clear (in some instances) as many books on food sensitivity lead one to believe. This is possibly due to a number of factors, not the least being that following such a rigorous regime requires an intelligent and highly motivated patient, as the disruption to lifestyle can be considerable in following an elimination diet. Also patients with illness due to foods often have a collection of vague symptoms, such as depression or fatigue, and find it exceptionally difficult to decide whether they are fatigued or depressed following any particular food. Therefore we find that elimination dieting is a useful technique, but with limited application due to the many practical problems which beset it.

Conclusion

All the testing methods mentioned in this chapter should be carried out within the setting of a clinical consultation. The findings must be interpreted in relationship to the patient's history, and the clinical experience and judgement of the practitioner are an integral part of this. In other words, the testing technique is only part of the story, and only provides a guide as to what the practitioner should recommend to the patient. If a range of sensitive foods is found and the patient avoids them and there is no clinical improvement, then as far as we are concerned the findings are irrelevant to the patient and we look at other possible causes of the problem.

Some of the techniques mentioned in this chapter can be carried out by any interested patient in their own home. The elimination dieting technique, the Coca pulse tests, and the sphygomanometer test are all easily carried out. If the results are not clear, then you are well advised to consult an appropriately qualified practitioner.

CHAPTER 7

Self-help in allergy

Clues to allergy

If you develop a runny, itchy nose in late May or early June, together with sneezing and sore eyes, it is not difficult to realize that you have hay fever due to pollen allergy. But in many other allergic problems there are clear clues in the same way which can lead to a suspicion that a problem is allergy-based, and often what the likely cause is. These clues come from several areas.

Season

Hay fever is the most obvious example, but further analysis of the exact timing of symptoms may identify what *type* of pollen is responsible. Grass pollen is usually at its height of production, depending on the weather, during June, whereas tree pollen occurs earlier. Occasionally we have seen symptoms for a very brief period in the summer, possibly as short as one week, and in this situation a single plant pollen, produced at this time, is responsible.

Moulds are also seasonal, but different species produce spores at different times all year round. Spores are released in response to wet weather, especially after a dry period, so autumn and spring are the worst seasons. Frost kills fungi, so a cold winter spell reduces the spores released, and people allergic to spores will notice their symptoms lessen when there are overnight frosts.

Another allergy showing seasonal variation is that to house dust and house dust mite. During the winter ventilation is reduced, central heating is switched on and we go out less. The warm, damp atmosphere in our houses produces ideal conditions for the house dust mite to thrive, and there is more human contact.

Timing

As well as contact with house dust being greater in winter, it is also greater at night. The mattress is a major source of dust, and close overnight contact may trigger worse symptoms. Asthma is commonly due to house dust, and the problem is therefore worse first thing in the morning and in winter.

Location

Where symptoms are worse can give clues which are as important as *when*. A condition which appears worse inside rather than outside is probably due to house dust or chemicals – if worse outside moulds or pollen are the likely cause. If symptoms seem worse at work, the possibility of chemicals or animal exposure must be considered. Clearly if there are pets in the house, and symptoms occur only at home, animal dander sensitivity is likely.

The location of the home may be important, particularly if the illness has worsened since a recent move, as shown by the following example.

CASE HISTORY

Sally was 5 when the family moved from a modern town house into a seventy year old house in the country. Some months later she developed a persistent cough, often in spasms so severe that they led to vomiting. Curiously, and to the parents inexplicably, she was better at school and when visiting friends in town – she had continued at her previous centre of town school.

It looked very much as if Sally's problems were due to a mould sensitivity, and this proved to be the case on testing. Her new home had some mould present and was near to wooded areas – both of which increased her mould exposure. A move was not needed. Appropriate desensitization and minimization of mould in the property provided the answer.

Occupation

Any occupation which exposes one to high levels of a possible allergen may lead to sensitization to that substance, with subsequent reaction even when exposed at low levels. Vets, for example, may become allergic to animals, and hairdressers to the chemicals they use. Even if they leave their job, contact through everyday items may perpetuate the problem. Clearly for clues from a person's occupation to be useful, a knowledge of what substances are encountered is essential.

Hobbies

Some people have unusual hobbies which put them in contact with possible sensitizing items. Amateur artists may develop a sensitivity to paint fumes, and evening electronic technicians may react to fumes from solder. In this area much the same information can be gained as from investigation of occupation.

Diet

People can develop symptoms due to recent dietary change, when there may have been an increase in some foods, due, for example, to changing to vegetarian habits. In addition food 'fads' may develop, causing a high intake of a particular food.

CASE HISTORY

Eric was a health fanatic. He jogged two miles daily, had weekly work-outs in the gym, and was a strict vegetarian. Naturally he was alarmed when he developed eczema, and had to seek help. Investigation of his diet was not adequately explored at the first consultation, and it seemed surprising that the only food which showed positive on testing was cauliflower. Eric then volunteered the information that he had recently been eating a whole cauliflower a day, as he had been informed (incorrectly) that cauliflowers were a 'complete food'. Treatment was easy, as cauliflower is not too difficult to avoid.

Frequently the food which is the underlying cause of a problem is a food to which the individual is almost addicted. Indeed, if there are no means available for testing, the most effective way of identifying an allergenic food is to ask 'what food would be most missed' – as there is often a craving for the food which is, in fact, harmful.

'DIY' diagnosis of allergies

The self-diagnosis of allergies is far from easy and not without risk. From a practical point of view it can only be done with allergenic substances which it is possible to avoid such as foods, but even then diagnosis is difficult and not always correct.

As will be mentioned in Chapter 9 there are some foods, containing the same chemical, to which a patient will be sensitive, but only if he/she takes them in the same meal or on the same day will problems occur. Each food, on its own, will probably not cause symptoms.

Bearing that in mind, the main methods of self-diagnosis in food allergy are explained below.

The food diary

This involves keeping a diary of foods ingested, together with a record of symptoms. If the sensitivity is to a single food (which is not usually the case) then this method will readily identify the offending item. It is also sometimes possible to show from a food diary that one item in the diet is taken more often and in larger quantity than average. As there seems to be a close association between intolerance and addiction – or at least a particular liking for a certain food – anything taken in excess may be the culprit.

CASE HISTORY

John had uncontrollable diarrhoea which often followed a meal. This was particularly difficult as his job involved entertaining potential clients, and there was little warning about his need to visit the toilet. A diary showed that it was usually after eating wheat products (including pasta) that his problems occurred. The diary also revealed that he had a high intake of beer, which of course contains wheat products. Although a wheat free diet proved difficult because of his craving for beer, his symptoms cleared, and he knows that if he gives in to his passion for ale he will pay the price!

Fast and reintroduction
This method of self-diagnosis is one frequently suggested, and often supervised by allergy practitioners. It is not only very demanding on the will-power of the patient, but is not without risk in terms of nutritional deprivation. The patient fasts for forty-eight hours, taking only spring water, and then introduces one food at a time, usually every alternate day, and notes when symptoms occur. The food most recently introduced is then considered to be the offending item.

A refinement of this method which is less demanding, is that instead of a total fast the subject is allowed one or two foods which rarely cause problems – lamb and pears commonly – during the first forty-eight hours.

This method is occasionally useful in identifying severe reactions, but if there are several foods to which the subject reacts which only cause problems if taken in combination, obviously this regime is inaccurate. In addition, the rigorous way in which the method has to be applied may lead to an obsession over minor symptoms not necessarily due to foods and an inadequate diet as a consequence.

The 'stone age' diet
This is a more acceptable form of the fast and reintroduction, in that a diet excluding the common items causing sensitivity is allowed, so such strict exclusion is not needed.

All foods are allowed except the following: all dairy products; all grains (wheat, rye, oats, corn, barley, rice); additives (colours, preservatives etc.); tea, coffee, alcohol; chocolate and refined sugar.

As has been mentioned, the common foods to cause problems are those taken on a daily basis, and the 'stone age' diet excludes these. After the diet has been maintained for two weeks, individual foods are reintroduced, again usually on alternate days, and any which cause symptoms to re-occur within twenty-four hours are avoided. Those which do not cause problems are incorporated into the diet.

The 'stone age' approach is probably the best initial strategy to take in self-diagnosis if a food sensitivity is suspected. It is not as rigid as the 'fast and reintroduction' method, and if symptoms persist it is still possible to change to one of the more rigid approaches.

A word of warning is essential regarding these dietary methods. If any strict diet is maintained for more than a few weeks, there may be an inadequate intake of essential vitamins and minerals, which itself could jeopardize health. It is vital to obtain professional advice from an ecologist or a dietician if the restricted diet is continued.

Food families

In the field of sensitivity and intolerance, not only is a person likely to be sensitive to a particular *type* of substance (i.e. animals or chemicals or foods), but with food sensitivity the problem may be within one group of foods. This group may be based on the food families, so that a person who is sensitive to potato may also react to other members of the potato family (tomato, pepper, tobacco, etc.), and someone who shows symptoms from taking oranges will probably react to other citrus fruits.

Because of this relationship, if a reaction to one food is discovered, it is probably wise to avoid other members of the same family initially. Detailed lists of foods and food families are provided in Chapter 20. Clearly some families, particularly cereals, are difficult to avoid as they are often 'hidden' in convenience foods and may constitute a major part of the diet. Reference to the diets in Chapter 20 will help to make sure they are avoided.

Food phenolics

As well as foods being related according to their family, or biological origin, there is a further relationship based on chemicals within foods. This is more fully discussed in Chapter 9, but some mention of it here is needed as there is a connection to food families.

In recent years some ninety chemicals which act as *natural* colours, flavours and preservatives in foods have been identified. Most of these are chemically similar (hence the name 'phenolics'). It is becoming clear that often these chemicals, rather than the foods themselves, can be the cause of the sensitivity. The link with food families is that sometimes foods in the same family have the same phenolics, but this is not always the case. Nicotine, for instance is contained in tomato, potato, and tobacco (all from one family), but is also in cheese, beef (another family), and chocolate and banana (which are unrelated). It may therefore be necessary to avoid all nicotine containing foods if there is a sensitivity to some of these items.

Three other important phenolic compounds are tyramine, caffeine and salicylates.

Tyramine is often the cause of migraine, and is present in high concentration in chocolate, red wine, cheese and oranges, which are recognised as triggers for some migraine sufferers. But it is also in eggs, tomatoes, spinach, aubergine and beef in lower amounts. If a sensitive person consumes several of these foods together the total 'dose' of tyramine may be as high as if they had consumed chocolate, and a migraine results.

Caffeine is a stimulant to the heart and nervous system. If sufficient is taken its effects may show in a non-sensitive person by producing heightened alertness, insomnia and palpitations. But in a sensitive person a very low dose may cause similar problems. Caffeine only occurs in tea, coffee, chocolate and cocoa.

Two salicylates occur in foods – methyl salicylate and acetyl salicylic acid. Their effects are similar, so the total salicylate level is the only aspect usually considered. They are in particularly high levels in fruits and some vegetables, corn and spices. Behavioural problems in children may be due to a high salicylate intake and a sensitivity to them.

Full lists of foods containing these phenolics can be found in Chapter 20.

Artificial additives

Much importance has been attached to the significance, in terms of health, of the effects of artificial colours, preservatives and other chemicals added to foods by the food industry. As these are non-natural it was felt that they were more likely to have adverse effects. This now does not appear to be the case as natural chemicals, mentioned above, can be equally damaging. Indeed some additives are positively beneficial – E300 is vitamin C.

There are some artificial additives though which should probably cause some concern.

Colours
The main potential culprits are the azo dyes and the coal-tar dyes, as they do not occur naturally. The numbers are E102, E104, E107, E110, E122, E123, E124, E127, E128, E129, E131,

E132, E133, E142, and E150. E150 is caramel, and products containing this often say 'caramel', not E150. Although caramel was originally a natural substance produced by the burning of sugar, it is now often made artificially. These colours are primarily used in confectionery foods and in convenience puddings.

Preservatives
E210 to E219 are the commonest cause of reactions. They are based on benzoic acid, which occurs naturally in fruits (especially berries) and may cause asthmatic symptoms. In addition the preservatives E250 and E251 (sodium nitrate and sodium nitrite) have been shown to change the haemoglobin in the blood, forming nitrosamines which are potentially cancer causing. These preservatives are mainly used in prepared meat products, such as sausages, and in alcoholic drinks.

Others
The flavour enhancer monosodium glutomate or E621 can cause the 'Chinese restaurant syndrome'. This name is used as Chinese foods often contain high levels of E621. In susceptible individuals the condition causes flushing, palpitations and tightness of the chest. In asthmatics a full attack may be induced. E621 is found mainly in savoury convenience foods.

Sensitivities – some common questions answered

Will my sensitivities be life-long?
Usually the answer to this is no. If the offending food(s) are avoided for some months there develops a tolerance to them to the extent that they may be taken again. The time that this takes varies from one individual to another, and also depends on how strictly they have avoided the food. On average, if the avoidance is total, reintroduction is possible approximately nine months later. Desensitization (see Chapter 10) may reduce this time. But if the food is restarted too early, a new problem rather than the previous symptoms may appear.

CASE HISTORY

Jane had severe eczema from the age of 2, and she was now 25. A careful history and testing showed that there was a sensitivity to milk, milk products, and beef. She avoided these rigorously, and in three months the eczema improved. After six months she became irritated by the social restrictions imposed by the diet, and started taking dairy products again. She was encouraged that there was no recurrence of the eczema, but as her intake increased she developed asthma. Her milk sensitivity was still present, but displayed itself with another illness.

It is unlikely that someone who has been sensitive to a food will ever be able to take it to the extent that they did previously – but a moderate intake is almost certainly possible.

What causes sensitivities to develop?
This is a complex question and one which is not, as yet, fully understood. It seems that heavy exposure to a particular agent to which one can become allergic makes it likely that a sensitivity to that substance may develop and appear later in life. But why this should affect some individuals and not others is not clear. It is likely that the presence of a dysbiosis (see Chapter 15) or candida (Chapter 14) predisposes a patient to the development of food sensitivity and this may have to be corrected to prevent further allergies developing.

CASE HISTORY

Merle was a West Indian immigrant, who came to the UK in her teens. When she was in her forties she developed irritable bowel syndrome, with abdominal pain, wind and diarrhoea. This was found to be due to an intolerance of corn (maize), and avoidance relieved the symptoms. It was later found that Merle had had a high intake of maize in childhood, as this is the staple cereal in Jamaica, which had sensitized her to later exposure.

How long will I have to avoid foods to which I am sensitive?
This varies from person to person, but on average will be around nine months. However if the avoidance has not been complete it will be longer. As a rule of thumb, for every time the diet is broken it will be another three days before the food can be introduced – so if 'cheating' on the diet is twice a week, the sensitivity may continue permanently.

Can I stop my doctor's treatment?
It is generally inadvisable to stop orthodox treatment, as it takes some time for the benefits of a diet to develop. In the intervening period there may be a worsening of the problem if medication is stopped. However, it is usually possible to *slowly* reduce – and possibly stop – medication after a few weeks of dietary restriction.

Will I get more sensitivities?
This depends on whether there is an underlying problem. Other conditions may make development of other sensitivities more likely, and these may have to be treated. But if overall health is otherwise good, new allergies are no more likely than in any other person.

What can I do if I am sensitive to so many things I can't avoid them all?
Allergies can be divided into two broad groups – those you can avoid (such as foods), and those you can't (such as dust and moulds). Sensitivity to the latter group needs desensitization approaches (see Chapter 10). If a person is sensitive to a large number of foods desensitization may again be needed, either to the food or to the phenolic responsible.

Self-diagnosis of food sensitivities is fraught with problems unless a very limited number of foods is involved. Not only may deficiencies of minerals and vitamins develop due to a restricted diet, but there is always the danger that coincidental symptoms may be attributed to a particular food, when there is some quite unrelated cause. This can end up with the potential patient becoming neurotic about their diet to an extreme. It is not unknown for such an approach to end up as a psychological eating disorder, rather than a problem in the ecological field, and this possibility should be borne in mind.

CHAPTER 8

Non-food sensitivity

There is a wide range of substances to which allergic individuals react which are not foods. These cover four main areas:

Airborne substances such as dust, dust mite, feathers, hair from cats, dogs, rabbits, etc.
Pollens.
Moulds and fungi.
Chemicals.

Sensitivity to dust, dust mite and animal hair

The most common symptoms these sensitivities produce are a persistently runny nose accompanied by sneezing (known as perennial or chronic rhinitis), sore itchy eyes, asthma and more rarely eczema.

Usually the reaction to animal fur is obvious, and the best treatment is to stop exposure to cats or dogs or whatever animals are involved. Desensitization using a dilution of a solution of the animal fur (the Miller technique), is another possibility if it is not possible to limit exposure.

CASE HISTORY

Jane is a vet who became sensitive to cats. This made it very difficult to continue her small animal practice. She had persistent itching, sneezing and running eyes on coming into contact with cats. Desensitization using a dilution of cat fur solution worked very well for her and allowed her to continue in her job.

Sensitivity to feathers, house dust and house dust mite is more difficult to diagnose, but it must be considered, particularly in asthma. Again desensitization is a useful approach, but a number of measures can be taken in the house, and certainly in the room where the asthmatic patient sleeps. They are as follows:

1. Get rid of carpets and soft furnishings in the bedroom.
2. Use a negative ioniser to get rid of as many dust particles from the atmosphere as possible.
3. Wrap the mattress in polythene.
4. Clean the room thoroughly every day when the occupant is out.
5. Do not use feather duvets or feather pillows.
6. In some instances, if patients are very sensitive to house dust mite it is possible to use a paint which contains an insecticide which will kill the house dust mite.
7. Use an anti-dust mite spray.

Pollen sensitivity

This is usually very obvious to diagnose, and it produces hay fever. In some patients this can be accompanied by asthma. There is usually a clear association between the pollen count and symptoms, but in severe cases symptoms can start as early as March and go on until late November. Generally speaking the season is from mid May until the end of July.

Limiting exposure to trees, grass or flowers, or all three, is one way of dealing with this, but this is not always practical. The best approach is to desensitize using dilutions of specific pollens, again using the Miller technique, or homoeopathic preparations using mixed pollens. A study published in the *Lancet* in October 1986 looked at using mixed pollens in the 30C potency (this refers to the specific dilution of the pollens in the homoeopathic preparation) in order to desensitize patients who were suffering from hay fever. This was a carefully conducted double blind controlled study, and showed that the homoeopathic preparation was significantly effective in relieving symptoms of hay fever. This is most interesting, in that firstly it validates the concept of homoeopathic dilution and secondly provides a useful treatment for hay fever.

Our experience is that homoeopathic desensitization, which should strictly be termed isopathic (iso means same, homoeo means similar) works well. We are in effect recommending the use of a homoeopathic pollen for a pollen sensitivity, therefore it is the same substance which is given isopathically and not a similar substance as in classical homoeopathy. Our clinical findings are that the isopathic preparations give different clinical results, and in some patients much better clinical results, than using the Miller technique. The mechanisms involved in both isopathy and the Miller technique are unknown. It is possible that they may have strong similarities however, as both utilize the concept of 'minimal dose therapy', but in slightly different ways, and with different methods of dilution, preparation and dosage.

CASE HISTORY

of desensitization with the Miller method

Ronald is a 68 year old farmer. Every spring and summer for some twenty years he has had severe hay fever, so that he was not able to carry out his normal work. On testing him he was sensitive to a wide range of grass pollens, flower pollens, tree pollens and he was desensitized to them. He responded partially to this approach, and on retesting it was found that he was also very sensitive to rape seed flowers. He was then desensitized to rape seed flower, and he remains symptom free providing he takes the desensitizing drops at least three times a day, and in some cases hourly, when the pollen count is particularly high. If he stays indoors all day, he rarely needs any drops. He has to start his drops in April and continue them right through until August. Each season, at the beginning of April, he has to have his desensitization end points worked out for the forthcoming season.

Mould and spore sensitivity

Sensitivity to moulds and spores is very widespread indeed, and some informed estimates have calculated that nearly 40% of the population in Britain react in some way to moulds and spores. Spores are released into the air at certain times of the year by fungi. For example, in the autumn, walking in damp woodlands reveals many different species of mushroom appearing between the leaves, which are discharging billions of spores into the atmosphere. At certain times of the year there are peaks so far as levels of spores in the atmosphere are concerned. The most marked peak is in the autumn, and there is a lesser peak in the spring.

Moulds and spores are more common in damp climates, and also in certain geographical areas such as low lying areas surrounded by trees and with nearby ponds or rivers. Extensively insulated houses are much more prone to mould growth than drafty airy Victorian types of houses. We commonly come across patients who develop persistently runny noses, asthma or eczema on moving into a new, well insulated house. Anybody with a family history of allergies should be careful if they are considering moving into such a house, even if it does save money on the heating bills.

The most common spores to which we are exposed are a number of species of airborne yeasts. These are followed by a number of other species with magnificent Latin names, the most common being sporobolomyces alternaria, cladosporum herbarum, penicillin species and species of aspergillus.

Of all the airborne substances, spores produce the most marked, and in some instances very serious, clinical symptoms. In some asthmatics these symptoms can be life threatening. We have also seen a number of patients with severe rheumatism, causing such marked pain in the limbs that the patient is confined to a wheelchair. Sensitivity to moulds and spores is responsible for some cases of eczema and can cause very severe eczema indeed. Mould and spore sensitivity can also produce chronic rhinitis, in which the patient complains of a runny stuffed-up nose. Other more uncommon symptoms include depression. Any history of a symptom that gets better in hot dry weather and worse in damp weather, almost always indicates that spore sensitivity is an important feature, and this is where treatment ought to be directed. It is particularly important to note whether symptoms improve on taking a holiday in a hot dry country such as Southern Spain. This is probably the best indicator from the history as to whether moulds and spores are involved.

Patients who have candidiasis (see Chapter 14), nearly always react to moulds and spores as candida is itself a spore. Spores are notoriously allergenic, and have outer coatings simply bristling with antigens to which the body reacts strongly.

Treatment involves eliminating damp, and this may mean calling in an architect. Adequate ventilation can be very important in keeping the house damp free. In very severe cases it may be necessary to consider moving house, or in the most severe cases even moving to a hot dry climate.

From a practical point of view Miller dilution desensitization for moulds is the only viable option. Very severely affected patients, particularly those with eczema, need to have a high potency isopathic preparation of specific moulds made up specially for them. The action of these preparations seems to be different from the Miller dilutions. Some patients, notably some with very severe eczema, do not respond to the Miller mould dilutions and often are made worse by them, but respond remarkably well to the correct isopathic potency of the relevant moulds. If you have mould sensitivity it is important to contact a practitioner who has a wide range of moulds in dilutions available for treatment.

Chemical sensitivity

Chemical sensitivity is becoming an increasingly important aspect of environmental medicine. The existence of chemical sensitivity was first noted by an American doctor, Dr. Albert Rowe, in the 1930s. He noticed that some of his patients reacted to apples which had been sprayed with pesticides, but not to ones taken from unsprayed orchards. This was the beginning of a growing awareness that pesticides, weedkillers and herbicides are potentially harmful to many people. These are not the only environmentally harmful chemicals, however, and many seemingly innocuous hydrocarbon products which all of us have in our homes are deadly poisonous to some people.

This area of environmental medicine is much more difficult to diagnose clinically with anything like the accuracy of specific food sensitivities, as often the patient has little knowledge as to whether he or she is exposed to a multitude of airborne chemicals. A testing method of some sort is essential to be able to identify and manage chemical sensitivity effectively.

Generally speaking, chemical sensitivities go hand in hand with food sensitivity. In some patients the chemical and hydrocarbon sensitivity predominates over the food sensitivity, in others foods are more important. It is usually possible to sort out the majority of environmental problems concentrating on foods alone, but unfortunately this situation is changing, particularly for the most sensitive people. For these it is necessary to unravel the tangle of chemical exposure in order to achieve a reasonable clinical result.

The outlook for the future is bleak as there are no signs that hydrocarbon, pesticide, food additive and aerosol propellant pollution is decreasing. Most chemical sensitivities are to hydrocarbons, particularly petrol, diesel and gas.

Hydrocarbon sensitivity

People with hydrocarbon sensitivity often complain of what the Americans describe as 'brain fag'. This is an intermittent state of varying severity (depending on the level of exposure) of mental confusion, poor memory, slurring of speech and a general dulling of all the senses, particularly sight. These symptoms can be caused by other sensitivities, but they are most commonly associated with hydrocarbons.

The clue as to whether the patient is sensitive to these substances comes from the history: for example, the patient who goes to sleep when sitting in front of a gas fire or near to a mobile calor gas heater, but not when sitting in front of an electric fire; the patient who suffers from car sickness; the motorist who constantly has to fight extreme fatigue when motorway driving; all this points to hydrocarbon sensitivity. Usually these people have an acute ability to smell even minute amounts of these fumes, but some of the most severely affected eventually lose any sense of smell as far as these hydrocarbons are concerned.

The best approach in dealing with these problems is to minimize exposure. This means getting rid of gas stoves and gas fires, while for petrol sensitive patients travelling in the front of the car where fumes are less marked can be helpful. A filter fitted to the car heater is also worth considering, as an unfiltered heater simply blows other vehicles' exhaust fumes into the car. Some Japanese cars have these fitted as a standard item.

Patients who react strongly to gas may need to go to the lengths of having all the gas pipes as well as gas boilers, cookers and fires removed from the house. Even pans and other utensils that have been used on a gas stove may need to be removed. This might sound like taking things too far, but any doctor who has been confronted by severely gas sensitive patients will be the first to concur with the usefulness of such apparently draconian advice.

Desensitization is clearly useful in these patients, as it means that they are able to cope with that level of exposure which is beyond their control. Many people cannot afford the measures suggested to create an environmentally safe haven for themselves. Desensitization can be a more manageable alternative for these people, although we have some doubts as to whether this is the best approach in the long term. Hydrocarbon sensitive people are advised to use electric heating instead of oil or gas fired central heating, even though the boiler may be situated outside the house.

CASE HISTORY

Joan is 36, and complains of headaches, confusion, poor memory, inability to concentrate. All these symptoms wax and wane and are much worse when she is at work. Her mental symptoms are classical 'brain fag' as described by the American clinical ecologists. She has been working in a garage as a secretary for some ten years and began to notice her symptoms after she had been working there for three years. During these ten years she has had two babies, and after each pregnancy her symptoms have become more persistent and more severe. She now notices that she reacts strongly to perfumes and to anything which is sprayed from an aerosol can. The most recent symptom is that she has been reacting to her packed lunch, which she takes to work in a tupperware plastic box. The sandwiches she eats now give her headaches and it seems to make no difference as to what is in them. In her family, her grandfather had asthma, and an aunt had irritable bowel syndrome.

This lady has some degree of allergic family history and she is working in a situation where there is high exposure to hydrocarbon fumes (petrol and diesel largely). With each pregnancy she has become more debilitated, and has not regained her previous state of health, in other words her immune reserve is smaller after the pregnancies than it was before she had any babies. She is gradually beginning to react to hydrocarbon derivatives such as perfumes and volatile plastics (this explains why she reacts to the sandwiches packed in the tupperware container).

Joan did only moderately well on desensitizing her to petrol, diesel, plastics and other hydrocarbon derivatives, because her exposure at work was so great that desensitization alone could not cope with this. She was helped considerably by appropriate nutritional therapy with carefully chosen vitamin and mineral replacement, and complex homoeopathy largely directed at the liver. In the end it was only possible to make her symptom free by getting her to change her job, which she did. She has had no symptoms since and is able to tolerate filling her own car with petrol without any symptoms.

Hydrocarbon derivatives
Substances derived from hydrocarbons are legion, and often patients who are sensitive to gas, petrol and diesel are also sensitive to many hydrocarbon derivatives. This covers a large group of substances. The main ones are:

Paint	Wax candles
Varnish	Coal fires
Solvent	Air freshener
Cleaning fluid	Deodorant
Lighter fuel	Disinfectant, especially
Propellant in aerosol sprays	pine-scented
Coal-tar soap	Cosmetics
Detergent	Perfume
Polish	Sponge rubber

Multiple chemically sensitive patients should be advised to avoid all these items. Hypo-allergenic all-purpose cleaning materials are now made by several companies, and these products are becoming more widely available through health food shops. We are often resistant to the idea of stopping the use of cosmetics and perfumes, but as many are hydrocarbon derivatives the results in terms of improved health are often gratifying.

Air pollution
Air pollution is becoming increasingly widespread. Admittedly it has improved in some particularly bad areas since clean air legislation has been introduced in many countries, but overall the situation is appalling. It is well within recent memory that

the notorious London smogs killed thousands of people. Such smogs are now more typical of parts of Eastern Europe, particularly Poland and Czechoslovakia. Air pollution is a major cause of many lung and heart diseases.

A major constituent of air pollution is vehicle exhaust fumes, consisting of a wide range of volatile organic compounds. In the presence of sunlight nitrogen oxides and sulphur dioxide undergo photochemical conversion to ozone, sulphuric acid and nitric acid gas. So far as people are concerned the main problem results from the transformation of gaseous sulphur dioxide (SO_2) into sulphuric acid (H_2SO_4), which is catalysed by various metals within water droplets in polluted air at relatively low temperatures. Various methods have been tried to counteract this and the only promising result has come from ammonia bottles with wicks that were placed in hospital wards in an attempt to neutralize the acid aerosols formed by sulphuric acid.

Because ammonia produced in the mouth appears to protect against the effects of acid air, it has been pointed out that this was one good reason why children in polluted areas should avoid lemonade, or acid sweets as this neutralizes the protective ammonia.

Recent research has now questioned whether increasing concentration of air pollutants may be linked to the increasing incidence and severity of some types of allergies. For example, in some countries including America, Australia, France and Britain, death rates from asthma have increased by 50% within the past ten years. It has been postulated that increased exposure to airborne allergens may be responsible. It has also been noticed that there has been a sharp increase in the incidence of hay fever, not affecting people living in country areas particularly, where the pollen exposure is highest, but interestingly those people living in urban environments who are exposed to high levels of air pollution. Diesel fumes seem to be particularly important. There can be no doubt also that high levels of certain air pollutants make asthma worse. The only reasonable reading of these findings is that if you have asthma, or severe hay fever, or even a family history of these illnesses, then it is worthwhile considering firstly moving to a non-urban countrified area, and if things are bad enough, attempting to work also in a non-polluted, non-urban environment.

Lastly, there is evidence that smoke particles are impregnated with polyaromatic hydrocarbons, and animal studies show that these are carcinogenic. The message is clear, if you are allergic avoid polluted environments. Desensitization is only a stop-gap measure, and will not remove any carcinogenic risks from air pollution.

Plastics
Articles made from hydrocarbon derivatives, particularly plastics, can affect hydrocarbon sensitive patients. Soft plastics of all types should be avoided. Storing food in tupperware-type containers will contaminate the food for these sensitive patients – glass storage jars are the safest method of food storage. Hard plastics such as bakelite are usually safe as they do not give off fumes in the same way that polythene does. Some people react to plastic glasses with sore, running eyes and irritation of the eyelids. These people should obtain steel rimmed glasses with the lenses free of plastic coating.

Synthetic clothing
Severely hydrocarbon sensitive patients should also take steps to avoid all close contact with clothing made of nylon and similar materials, since these are derived wholly or in part from hydrocarbons. This therefore means dressing in clothes made from natural materials such as wool or cotton; in practice these can be difficult to obtain and a mixture of 70% wool or cotton with the rest being a man-made fibre is often the purest that can be obtained, but it is well worth searching to obtain pure wool or pure cotton garments. This sort of attention to detail can produce enormous dividends in the health of these patients.

Phenol
Phenol, or carbolic, rather like hydrocarbons, is a ubiquitous chemical. It is contained or used in the manufacture of the following:

Herbicides	Petrol (traffic fumes)
Pesticides	Dye
Bakelite	Photographic solutions
Moulded articles like	Preservative in allergy
telephones	antigen solutions
Synthetic detergent	Epoxy and phenoxic resins

Aspirin and other drugs
Nylon
Polyurethane
Explosives

Casing of electric wiring and
cables
Perfume

Formalin
The use of formalin is widespread and people are often sensitive to it. It is found in the following:

Traffic fumes
Glue and cement
Matches
Synthetic foam rubber
All propellants (sprays)
Fabric softener/conditioner
Orthopaedic casts
Hospital sick rooms
Surgical instrument cleaning
Manufacture of vitamins A
and E
Textile dyes, permanent-press
treatment, wrinkle-resisting
treatment, mildew-proofing,
water-repellant treatment,
shrink-proofing, moth-
proofing, stretch fabrics
Paper manufacture
Newsprint
Photography and
photographs
Milk products, including
powdered cream
Antiperspirant

Disinfectant
Antiseptic for dentures
Mouthwash
Nail polish
Toothpaste
Insecticides
Fertilizers
Tanning agent in tanning of
animal skins
Soft plastics
Germicidal soap
Detergent
Shampoo
Hair setting lotion
Air deodorants
Waste incineration
Building materials, concrete,
plaster, wallboard, synthetic
resin, wood veneer, wood
preservative
Cavity-wall insulation
Manufacture of antibiotics
Polluted air

Chemical pollution of meat
Practically all meat available in the average butcher's shop has been intensively reared and generally contains trace levels of antibiotics and in some cases other drugs, which have been given to the animals. Some very sensitive patients react to meat, and indeed to many foods, simply because of the contaminants that these foods contain. Our experience has convinced us that if these patients can obtain and eat organic, uncontaminated food they can often tolerate these foods with no reaction at all.

All of these food sources are relatively expensive. Patients who are unable to buy organic meat would be well advised to become vegetarian and grow as much of their own food as possible. Unfortunately even this is not entirely free from danger, as a recent study on lead levels in vegetables has shown that vegetables, particularly brassicas, grown within a ten mile radius of central London contain unacceptably high levels of lead due to atmospheric pollution. Perhaps the abolition of lead in petrol may help to reverse this sad situation.

Food colourants

The addition of colourants to processed foods is common practice, as this makes the food look attractive and therefore more saleable. Frozen peas often look almost luminous; orange squash looks bright orange. Whilst looking attractive, this can play havoc with some patients: disorders of the nervous system, particularly hyperactivity in children, have been closely associated with reaction to colourants, especially tartrazine (an orange colourant). Tartrazine has also been associated with childhood asthma. These connections have been recognized in the United States where tartrazine is banned, but ironically many children's medicines contain added colourant, often making the sensitive child worse. Parents of such children would be well advised to ask for colourless medicine.

Colourants probably have a pharmacological (drug-like) effect on sensitive individuals as they seem to have a predilection for nerve synapses, the 'relay stations' in the nervous system where one nerve ends and another begins. Highly complex neurochemical reactions occur at synapses and these processes are very sensitive to modulation by any chemical which happens to be around. Colourants seem to be a group of compounds which can modulate synaptic transmission of nerve impulses, often facilitating this transmission and therefore producing hyperactivity. The only effective treatment for colourant sensitivity is avoidance.

Artificial colourants are commonly added to such food as crème de menthe, glacé cherries, coloured ice creams, coloured sweets, some cheeses, butter, margarine, artificial orange squash, cola and other coloured soft drinks, and many processed foods.

Drugs

Sensitivity to drugs is more widespread than the medical profession likes to think. Recent evidence has found a possible connection between patients who react to many drugs and enzyme deficiency. This means that some people, because of enzyme deficiency, deal with drugs in a different way to others. Unfortunately this does not tell us how to prevent it happening. It is therefore wise for patients with multiple sensitivities to take as few drugs as possible, and to obtain treatment using an alternative therapy which has fewer side-effects.

It is important to maintain a balanced view when discussing modern drug therapy, as its 'popular face' leads one to suspect that all drug therapy is bad. This is far from the truth, as many modern drugs are life-savers – antibiotics and anticoagulants being two obvious examples. Many others are obviously harmful and potentially lethal. It is important for patients to receive medical advice which reflects an unprejudiced view of both alternative and modern drug approaches.

Tap water

Tap water contains a vast array of chemicals, the most dangerous being lead, cadmium and nitrates (derived from fertilizers used in agriculture). Upper limits allowed are clearly defined for many of these chemicals, yet in our experience an alarming number of patients with illness due to environmental factors react to tap water. This raises the question as to what upper limits of safety means; safe for whom? Certainly not the sensitive patient. Most people reacting to tap water do so after drinking it; a few also react when they wash in it, particularly patients with eczema. The treatment is to avoid tap water and drink bottled spring water. Filtering tap water is another possibility, and this can be done through a simple cheap water filter or a more sophisticated filter such as reverse osmosis filters.

Soaps and detergents

These are often a forgotten part in environmentally caused illness. An obvious piece of advice is that biological washing powders should be avoided, since they can cause eczema in some patients. All coal-tar derived soaps should be looked upon with suspicion, as must any scented soap, particularly pine scented.

Tobacco smoke
Nearly all chemically sensitive patients are sensitive to tobacco smoke. If they smoke themselves they should make a real effort to stop. They should also avoid crowded, smoke-filled places such as pubs, some restaurants and smoking compartments in trains.

What can be done for the multiply chemically sensitive patient?

Avoidance
The best approach is avoidance and the creation of a safe haven both at home and work. A useful additional idea is the use of a portable air filter.

Desensitization
Miller type desensitization is an important means of helping people with chemical sensitivity. The most common chemicals we give desensitization drops for are gas, petrol, diesel, paint fumes (terpenes), ethanol, phenol, formalin, butane and propane.

Isopathic desensitization
Using principles of homoeopathy, high dilutions of the chemicals to which a patient is sensitive can encourage desensitization. Thus a 30C or a 200C dilution of the chemical to which a patient is sensitive taken once daily or, in the latter instance, on alternate days may result in a reduction in sensitivity. This method can be as effective as Miller desensitization, and has the advantage of once daily administration. The homoeopathic dilution is not as specific to the patient as in the Miller technique. This means isopathic dilutions are often better tolerated than Miller desensitization. Ideally both techniques should be available, so that the more effective and best tolerated approach can be selected for each individual patient.

CHAPTER 9

Sensitivity to common chemicals in foods

As previously touched on, it is now recognized that sensitivity to foods may be due to a sensitivity to particular natural chemicals within those foods. It should be emphasized that these compounds are naturally occurring, not artificially added during production, and act as natural colours, preservatives and flavourings to the foods.

Some, though by no means all, of these chemicals are based on the benzene ring, which is a ring of six carbon atoms.

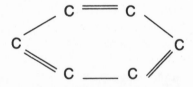

It is because of this structure that the chemicals are known collectively, but slightly incorrectly, as the phenolic chemicals – this ring is the basic structure of phenol. The variation between each phenolic chemical is in the make-up of the different branches from each carbon atom. Among the chemicals in this group are many of the body's messengers such as neurotransmitters and hormones. Indeed, as will be seen, some of these chemicals (for example oestrogen and serotonin) are also present in some foods. Sensitivity to these 'phenolic' substances is also clinically important.

If a patient is sensitive to a number of different foods, it may be possible to identify a common phenolic chemical present in these foods, and it is this which is in fact causing symptoms in the patient. With some of these chemicals it is now recognized that the reaction by the patient is not a truly allergic one, but is an intolerance or sensitivity. The patients can take up to a certain level of this particular chemical, and hence foods which contain it, but if they exceed their own individual sensitivity level they develop symptoms. The effect is probably therefore a cumulative pharmacological, or drug-like, effect, not a sensitivity in the way previously discussed. It is for this reason that it is often difficult for patients to identify foods to which they are sensitive, as they may find that individual foods cause no problems, but when foods containing the same phenolic are taken together their total tolerance is exceeded and they therefore develop symptoms.

A simple example of this would be a patient who is sensitive to nicotine. Nicotine is not only present in tobacco, but also in tomato, potato, cheese, banana, beef, chocolate and malt. Patients may find that they are able to take an individual food from this list, but when several foods are taken at once their tolerance of nicotine is exceeded and they then develop symptoms.

This situation is well recognized with the chemical caffeine, which as most people know is present in tea, coffee and chocolate. Most people can tolerate a few cups of coffee a day, but if intake is excessive then the drug-like effects of caffeine – stimulation and insomnia – develop.

The phenolic chemicals which have so far been identified in food are give below; * indicates compounds commonly causing toxic or allergic problems.

Phenolic compounds present in foods

Acetaldehyde	Acetone	Adenine
Aflatoxins	Amino benzoic acid	Amino butyric acid
Amygdalin	Anethole	Anisole
Apiol	Aspargin	Benzaldehyde
Benzoic acid*	Benzyl alcohol	Butylated-hydroxyanisole
Butylated hydroxy-toluene	Butyric acid	Caffeic acid
Caffeine*	Camphor	Capsaicin*
Carotene	Caryophylline	Chalcone
Choline	Chlorogenic acid	Cineol
Cinnamaldehyde	Cinnamic acid	Coniferyl
Coumarin	L-Dopa	Dopamine
Ellagic acid	Eugenol	Folic acid
Formaldehyde*	Furfural	Gallic acid

Genistein	Glutamine	Hesperetin
Histamine	Indole	Isoascorbic acid
Limonene	Linalool	Malvin*
Menadione	Menthol	Methylsalicylate*
Naringenin	Nicotine*	Noradrenaline
Octopamine	Oestrogen	Phenylalanine
Phenylisothio-cyanate*	Phloridzin	Pinene
Piperine	Piperonal	Progesterone
Putrescine	Pyridine	Pyrrole
Rutin	Safrole	Serotonin
Thujone	Thymol	Thymine
Tryptamine	Tyramine*	Tyrosine
Uric acid	Vanillin	Vanillylamine
Xanthine*		

It is now known that individuals who show sensitivity to some of these chemicals are lacking in enzymes which break down the compounds prior to excretion. This is particularly the case with tyramine, which is a common cause of migraine headaches. Many migraine sufferers have been shown to have a deficiency of the enzyme in the liver which clears tyramine from the blood stream, and therefore if large amounts of tyramine are taken in the diet a migraine can result. However, as so many foods contain tyramine in varying concentration it is difficult to identify the particular causative items.

The situation therefore is rather like that which has been referred to elsewhere, the 'barrel' concept. Patients who are sensitive to a particular chemical can be envisaged as having a barrel within their system which takes on board the particular chemical to which they react, till the barrel is filled to overflowing, when symptoms will develop. If the diet is restricted so that the particular phenolic chemical is not ingested to the same extent, the barrel will not overflow and symptoms will therefore not develop.

An important further development of this idea is to envisage that the more the barrel overflows the smaller it becomes, in other words if symptoms occur frequently the patient can tolerate smaller and smaller amounts of the chemical. However, if the diet is restricted to the extent that the barrel does not overflow, then the barrel will, over a period of months, enlarge its capacity. The patients will then be able to take larger quantities of the food to which they were previously sensitive, but in the case of phenolic chemicals it is likely that some degree of sensitivity will be life-long although eventually the diet may have to be restricted only marginally.

Phenolic compounds causing sensitivity problems

The following chemicals, together with details of foods in which they occur, are commonly encountered causes of problems.

Tyramine

As mentioned above, tyramine is a potent cause of migraine. If a normal patient, who does not suffer from migraine, was injected with a sufficient quantity of tyramine he/she would probably develop migraine, as it causes spasm of the arteries within the brain. Migraine sufferers are often unable to metabolize tyramine and it therefore builds up to dangerous levels in the bloodstream.

A large number of foods contain tyramine, but it is in particularly high concentration in those foods which have long been recognized as a cause of migraine – cheese, chocolate, red wine. Tyramine is also present in high levels in other foods such as hung game, liver and yeast extract. Smaller concentrations of tyramine are found in spinach, banana, eggs, chicken, oranges and continental smoked sausages. If sufficient of these latter foods are taken, tyramine ingestion may therefore also be enough to trigger a migraine.

Nicotine

The foods containing nicotine have been mentioned on p. 101. Nicotine can also be a migraine causing agent. In addition, nicotine can be associated with anxiety and palpitations, symptoms which often occur together.

Phenylisothiocyanate

Recent research suggests that this chemical may be causative in inflammatory bowel conditions such as ulcerative colitis and Crohn's disease. Phenylisothiocyanate (or PITC for short) is a highly caustic substance, which if applied to skin in neat form would cause ulceration. Avoidance of it is difficult as it is present both in dairy products and in soya beans, and soya milk is frequently used as an alternative to cow's milk.

PITC is in fact present in all beans, broccoli, Brussels sprouts, cocoa, chocolate, cow's milk, lamb, onion, peas, peppercorns, radish, tomato and turnip. In some patients with inflammatory bowel disorder total avoidance of these items has resulted in a dramatic improvement.

Salicylate

Aspirin is a salicylate, but it is often not realised that salicylates occur in foods as well, as methyl salicylate and acetyl salicylic acid. Sensitivity to salicylates is a common cause of hyperactivity in children. It has long been recognized that some hyperactive children respond to dietary restriction according to the Feingold diet, as proposed by Dr. Feingold in the 1960s. Although he was unaware of it at the time this is in fact a diet which reduces the intake of salicylates.

Salicylates are present in a very large number of foods, but are particularly prevalent in highly flavoured fruits and vegetables. The fact that nowadays children have a high intake of such foods, particularly in the form of fruit juices, may be one reason why hyperactivity appears to be on the increase.

As is so common in dietary sensitivity, the food to which the patient is reacting is often one which contains the phenolic to which they are sensitive. This is particularly true with salicylate sensitivity. A child who ingests large quantities of fruit juice, or tomato products, and is fond of cola drinks and strong mints, may well have a salicylate sensitivity.

Formalin

Sensitivity to formalin has been discussed in Chapter 8 as it is a chemical pollutant which is frequently encountered in the environment. It is a volatile compound, and therefore exists as a vapour given off by such substances as dyes, soaps, detergents, etc. However it is present in some foods (apple, asparagus, avocado, cherry, coffee, honey, cow's and goat's milk, mushroom, pineapple, yeast). Patients who are sensitive to formalin in the atmosphere may well also be sensitive to it in their diet and exclusion of the above items is essential for their full recovery.

Benzoic acid

Reaction to an over-intake of benzoic acid can also show as behavioural disturbance, particularly in children. Benzoic acid is a naturally occurring preservative, but is now also added, with its derivatives, to foods as an artificial preservative (numbers E210-E219 inclusive). It occurs naturally in most fruits, dairy products and tomatoes.

Malvin
Some patients have been known to be sensitive to malvin in that they demonstrate learning difficulties when exposed to large doses. Again it is a chemical mainly present in fruits, but also in vegetables and beet sugar (not cane sugar).

Nitrates
Whilst nitrates are not a phenolic compound, mention should be made of sensitivity to them at this point. Nitrates are increasingly found in our foods due to their use as a fertilizer, from where they get into ground water and hence into tap water. High levels are found particularly in radishes, lettuce, beetroot and beet sugar. Nitrates too can affect behaviour in children.

Hormones and neurotransmitters

Some of the chemicals mentioned in the list above are hormones. Others are chemicals which directly affect nerves and act as messengers in the body between nerve cells (neurotransmitters). A further development of the research on phenolic compounds has shown that irrespective of intake of these chemicals through foods, some conditions may be due to a hypersensitivity to these chemicals within our own bodies.

Premenstrual tension
Orthodox medicine considers that premenstrual tension is due to a lack of progesterone in the few days prior to the period. However, it seems possible that patients are not reacting to the progesterone which they are producing, and therefore reacting *as if* they were deficient. Techniques usually used for desensitization to these chemicals in the diet appear to actually *resensitize* the body to hormones and neurotransmitters, and can therefore be used to treat this condition without hormone replacement and the risks which this entails.

Menopausal problems

These can sometimes be helped by desensitization to oestrogen, and even if this is not totally effective it can often improve symptoms dramatically.

Epilepsy

Serotonin is a neurotransmitter, and some patients with epilepsy appear to be hypersensitive to it, so that instead of one or two nerve cells firing at its production a large number do this together, which initiates a fit. Desensitization to serotonin can therefore often help by reducing this reaction.

Enuresis (bed wetting)

Some patients with this problem show a sensitivity to one of the neurotransmitter phenolics, and may be helped by appropriate desensitization and/or avoidance.

Rather than testing a large number of foods and identifying the individual foods to which a patient is sensitive, it is possible to test by methods previously described a patient's reaction to individual phenolics. However it is usual to test foods first, from which a common phenolic chemical can often be identified. Thus if a patient who complains of migraine headache on testing shows sensitivities to cheese, chocolate, beef, bananas, orange and spinach, the practitioner would become suspicious that tyramine is involved, and will be able to test tyramine separately. This concept is of particular importance as it is then possible, instead of desensitizing the patient to each food individually, to desensitize to the one phenolic chemical.

Whilst the study of the reactions to phenolic chemicals is in its infancy, it is hoped that the possibilities demonstrated so far might become more widely used as an additional approach within the ecological field.

CHAPTER 10

The management of ecological illness

Once a clear diagnosis has been made of which foods and chemicals to avoid the battle is largely won. Treatment is either by avoidance of the offending items or by rotation dieting and/ or desensitization.

Food avoidance and rotation diets

The simplest approach is to exclude the sensitive foods from the diet. It is important to vary the remaining foods as much as possible, and the system for doing this is called rotation dieting. This means not eating one food within three days of having eaten it previously (a three day rotation) or sometimes within seven days (a seven day rotation). The longer the rotation, the more difficult the diet is to design. The idea of rotation dieting is to minimize the chances of developing sensitivity to new foods. The majority of food sensitive patients manage very satisfactorily on simple avoidance and rotation dieting, but in very sensitive patients this simple approach breaks down and desensitization along with homoeopathic treatment is essential.

As a general rule, once the foods to which the patient has been sensitive have been avoided for six to nine months, they can be carefully reintroduced into a rotation dieting plan. At this stage the average patient has developed tolerance to these foods, but if they are eaten with anything like the regularity they were before food avoidance, then masked sensitivity will develop again. Some food sensitivities appear to be fixed in that tolerance never develops. This is perhaps due to lack of essential enzymes in particular patients to cope with these foods. The best example is lactase deficiency for digesting milk and dairy products.

An example of a seven day rotation diet of a patient who is very sensitive to grains (wheat, oats and rye), pork, milk and dairy products

	Monday	Tuesday	Wednesday	Thursday	Friday	Saturday	Sunday
Meat:	Chicken	Beef	Pork	Lamb	Fish	Turkey	Game
Fruit:	Citrus	Berries	Banana	Pear	Plum	Apple	Kiwi, Mango
Vegetables:	Root	Leaf (Cabbage, Spinach etc.)	Peas	Beans	Potato	Tomato	Onion, Leek etc.
Cereal:	Wheat	Corn	Rice	Buckwheat	Oats	Millet	Rye
Dairy Products:	–	Cheese	–	–	–	Milk	–

Note that not more than one food to which the patient is sensitive – underlined – is taken on any particular day.

Some practitioners recommend rotating food families as well as individual foods: for example, potatoes and tomatoes belong to the same family and therefore should not be eaten within three days of each other on a three day rotation.

Desensitization

This has been described in some detail in Chapter 6. The principle is to find a dilution of the food or chemical or airborne substance to which the patient is sensitive which will switch their reaction to the relevant substance off. Generally speaking, the 'switch-off' is given in the form of drops. One drop is put under the tongue approximately ten minutes before exposure to the food, chemical or airborne allergen. In multiply sensitive individuals cocktails may be made containing mixtures of many food and chemical 'switch-off' drops. These patients usually need to take their drops regularly as they will suffer exposure to various irritants throughout the day.

Some practitioners recommend 'switch-off' by injection just beneath the surface of the skin, claiming that these produce a longer-lasting effect of two or three days, and they suggest that injections are more effective than sublingual drops. Sublingual drops only work for a few hours and therefore have to be taken at least three times daily if exposure to the food or chemical is occurring regularly; in some instances drops may have to be taken hourly if exposure is particularly heavy, such as to gas or petrol fumes. In our experience, injection just beneath the skin of 'switch-off' drops does produce longer lasting symptom relief than drops under the tongue. However, we have not found that injections into the skin are any more effective than sublingual drops. We therefore use the sublingual route exclusively as it is more convenient.

Methods of locating the 'switch-off' end point

A number of methods can be used to find the dilution which switches the patient's reaction off. The most commonly used is the intradermal injection technique described by Dr. Joe Miller. The ACR, electrical testing using the Vega apparatus or applied kinesiology can also be used.

The major disadvantages of the intradermal technique are that it is time-consuming (in our hands it takes approximately forty minutes to determine one end point) and that the symptoms it produces during a testing session can be difficult to reverse in very sensitive patients. We have known patients pass out on intradermal injection of substances to which they are sensitive. In one extreme case, one lady reacted to a mould in this way and remained unconscious for a day and a half until the appropriate end point was found. In this particular instance, managed by a colleague who very much favours the intradermal injection technique for finding the neutralization end point, she was maintained in fluid balance using an intravenous drip, and dilutions of the mould were successively placed under her tongue, and it was not until the 520th dilution that she came out of her comatose state! She came round within a few seconds. This is indeed an extraordinary finding, and it also vindicates the neutralization end point technique.

When finding the end points using the intradermal injection technique, and in fact this technique can also be carried out simply by putting the drops under the patient's tongue, the patient keeps a symptom diary, and ten minutes is left between giving each dilution. Any symptoms occurring are carefully noted in this diary, and the dilution which switches his or her symptoms off is also carefully noted. This is the 'switch-off' dilution.

The ACR, the Vegatest electrical method, and applied kinesiology methods for finding end points are all quick and do not cause symptoms in the patient except in the most sensitive cases. In these cases simply connecting them up to the substance to which they are sensitive can be enough to cause a reaction. This sort of reaction does occur only with the Vegatest, not if the ACR or applied kinesiology methods are used. This underlines how extremely sensitive some people are. In our view electrical testing is the most convenient method; and an end point can be determined in approximately three minutes using this technique. The disadvantage is that considerable skill on the part of the practitioner is needed.

Mechanism of action of desensitization

The mode of action of ecological desensitization is unclear. In our opinion an electrical mechanism of an ill-understood nature is involved as the 'switch-off' often occurs rapidly following a single drop under the tongue. It surprises us that this method of desensitization seems to be accepted uncritically by many doctors practising ecology, as it has many parallels with homoeopathy, the healing art which continues to attract derision from many doctors, including some ecologists.

Use of desensitization

Desensitization is useful for patients who cannot follow a strict diet due to pressures of a busy life or a difficult home environment. It is essential in patients who are so multiply sensitive that their safe diet is nutritionally inadequate. Desensitization at least allows these patients to expand their diets and thereby maintain adequate nutrition. Patients who are chemically sensitive, particularly to airborne chemicals, need desensitization if they are going to lead a reasonable existence in an urban environment where it is impossible to avoid petrol or diesel fumes. Desensitization offers some hope for these patients who, for reasons of job or family commitments, are unable to make sufficiently rigorous environmental changes to avoid exposure to airborne chemicals. The same applies to other airborne substances, particularly fungal spores and dust and dust mite.

Return of symptoms whilst taking desensitization drops

Some patients develop symptoms again after having been successfully 'switched-off' to the foods and chemicals or airborne substances to which they were sensitive. This is usually due to a change in the 'switch-off' point, but can be due to the development of another sensitivity. This means that patients on 'switch-off' drops need to have their end points checked periodically.

If injection into the skin is used to determine 'switch-offs' then this can be an expensive procedure. As yet none of these methods are commonly available within the NHS. Clearly, cheaper techniques such as the ACR, or electrical testing or muscle testing would be more suitable in a Health Service situation. However, none of these methods are credible enough in the eyes of conventional medicine. Perhaps further research will give them the respectability they need and they can then be incorporated into regular medical care.

For how long does desensitization need to be continued?

The average patient with ecological illness loses his sensitivities following a prolonged period of avoidance, usually in the order of two or three years. Desensitization under the tongue usually shortens this time to two years or even eighteen months in some cases, when often the patient can gradually come off drops and tolerate moderate intermittent exposure to the previously sensitive foods and chemicals.

Homoeopathic desensitization
It is possible to use an isopathic technique, in which the patient takes a potency of the substance to which he is sensitive. This works in certain patients, and in certain instances, particularly fungal spores, high potencies are required, which are then often only taken one drop every three or four days. In order to determine which potency is required (a whole range of potencies is needed to choose from), a testing technique of some sort must be used.

Disadvantages of desensitization
Desensitization is by no means always successful. The more sensitive the patient, the less likely it is that it offers a practical solution. Often in these patients end points change rapidly, and in some cases almost daily, so it becomes impractical to keep changing their medicines. Some patients on desensitization have an alarming tendency to develop more sensitivities, and in our experience desensitization may accelerate this tendency amongst the most sensitive patients. This therefore favours looking very carefully for underlying causes of the patient's multiple sensitive state. Chapters 13 to 17 look in detail at the most common of these underlying causes.

Enzyme potentiated desensitization (EPD)
This is a method for treating allergies which has been developed by Dr. Len McEwen, originally of St. Mary's Hospital Medical School, London, and latterly of the London Medical Centre. The method consists of placing a mixture of highly purified antigens, in very small doses indeed, with an enzyme called β-glucuronidase to potentiate the effect of the antigens mixed together with two other chemicals.

Although formerly the treatment was carried out through a technique involving slow absorption through a small area of abraded skin on the forearm, with the material held in place by a plastic slide retained by strapping for twenty-four hours, this method has now very largely been replaced by an intradermal injection in the same site. As the volume of fluid is similar to that used in the Miller technique the appearance of the site is similar, although it does not give rise to similar skin or systemic reactions at the time of the injection.

It is usual to apply a standard mixture of more than seventy allergens, in the hope that all the important ones have been included, so it is not essential to identify all the patient's sensitivities. The tendency to develop new sensitivities seen so often in sublingual desensitization is not apparent with this method. These factors give it obvious advantages over the 'switch-off' drop method.

Treatment is usually given monthly for three months, with booster doses every four months after that. The average patient with food sensitivities can expect to develop tolerance to his or her sensitive foods in six to twelve months from starting treatment – unlike desensitization drops, it does not work immediately. To date this method is not widely available and so far as we know is not offered within the NHS. Like sublingual desensitization it is much less useful in the patient with multiple sensitivities.

CHAPTER 11

The role of vitamins and minerals

Although this book is mainly concerned with illnesses caused by allergy and sensitivity, some information about the place of the essential chemicals in the diet is important. Readers may be tempted to restrict their diets (or be advised to by a practitioner), and this could result in too low an intake of some items, with resulting secondary illness.

It is important, when considering the part that vitamins and minerals have to play in health, to be aware of the subdivisions which exist with these chemicals. Some are known to be essential to health, whereas the role of others may not be essential. In addition, some vitamins and minerals may be toxic if taken in large quantities. Moderate intake is therefore essential, but excessive intake, as well as a deficient intake, may cause illness rather than prevent it.

Fundamentally these compounds divide into three groups.

1. Vitamins. The vitamins are a range of complex chemicals which are essential to normal healthy metabolism and the maintenance of life.

In order to be considered to be a vitamin the compound must only be available from the diet; cause specific symptoms when deficient; and those symptoms must be cured on administration of the vitamin.

This explains, to some extent, the apparently illogical numbering system – some compounds on discovery were thought to be vitamins, but later research demonstrated that they did not fulfill the criteria. Even now there are some chemicals designated as vitamins which do not strictly comply.

Vitamin D, for example, is produced in the body through the action of sunlight, and only in infants and those not exposed to sunlight is dietary intake necessary.

Vitamins are divisible into fat soluble and water soluble. This distinction is important as the fat soluble vitamins, if taken in excess, can rapidly become toxic as they are not easily excreted from the body. The water soluble vitamins, on the other hand, are normally rapidly excreted, usually via the kidneys, and overdosage is therefore not a risk unless taken in excessively high dose. Although the role of most vitamins is known, there are some for which this is not yet so. Some are known to be essential in animals, but their necessity in humans is open to question.

2. Essential minerals. These are elements, frequently metals, which are present in the body in small amounts, and which are essential to specific functions within the body. Some are fundamental to the structure of tissues (e.g. calcium in bone), whereas others are needed in enzyme processes for normal metabolism. Although the need for vitamins has long been established, the health effects of mineral deficiency are only just beginning to be recognized, and it would seem that they are probably as important as the vitamins for optimum health.

3. Trace elements. The human body contains minute traces, less than 0.01% of body weight, of some chemicals which *may* play a part in maintaining efficient functioning of the organism. The role of essential minerals is now largely established, but the way in which trace elements exert their effect is largely unknown.

Supplementation

There is much debate regarding the necessity or otherwise of regular vitamin and mineral supplementation to the diet. The problem is compounded by the fact that excessive intake of some vitamins and minerals can result in toxicity, causing illness, and that other factors, such as the individual diet and absorption may affect the levels in a particular person. Broadly speaking, supplementation can be considered in three distinct situations.

1. Supplements may be taken by a healthy individual to ensure that deficiency will not occur. Such supplementation should contain enough of the desirable vitamins and minerals to make certain that irrespective of any dietary restriction the daily intake for each vitamin and mineral is maintained. At the same time, the intake of those vitamins which are potentially

toxic should be at a level which will not cause toxicity, again irrespective of dietary habits.

2. The life style, occupation, age and health of an individual may make supplements of particular vitamins and minerals desirable. It is, for example, normal practice to give extra iron and folic acid during pregnancy, and there is also evidence that zinc intake should be increased in this condition. Children have higher requirements of calcium, and the elderly, because they often have inadequate dietary intake, may need supplements of vitamins C and B-complex. Also, many medications interfere with the absorption, or increase the excretion of vitamins. The contraceptive pill enhances the possibility of vitamin B6 deficiency, and diuretics increase the excretion of potassium and calcium. In this chapter, factors which may increase requirements are considered under each supplement.

3. It is becoming increasingly common to use very high doses of some vitamins as treatment in specific conditions. In particular, vitamin C can be given by intravenous infusion directly into the blood stream in a dose 250 times greater than the recommended daily intake in toxic conditions and infections. Some practitioners recommend high oral doses of vitamin E in heart conditions.

This area remains very controversial, mainly as the way in which it works is, at present, unknown. Nevertheless increasing numbers of doctors are using high dosage supplementation.

Recommended daily intake

Although there are published government recommended intakes for some vitamins, this does not cover all vitamins and only three minerals. In addition, it would seem that these levels may only be those which are necessary to prevent illness, not the level which is required for optimum health. For example, an intake of 60-100 mgm vitamin C a day will prevent the onset of scurvy, but to maintain adequate defences against infection, more than ten times this intake may be needed.

Vitamins

	Vit A micro-gram	Thiamin (B1) milligram	Riboflavin (B2) milligram	Niacin (B3) milligram	Vit C milligram	Vit D micro-gram
Boys:						
under 1	450	0.3	0.4	5	20	7.5
1	300	0.5	0.6	7	20	10
2	300	0.6	0.7	8	20	10
3-4	300	0.6	0.8	9	20	10
5-6	300	0.7	0.9	10	20	–
7-8	400	0.8	1.0	11	20	–
9-11	575	0.9	1.2	14	25	–
12-14	725	1.1	1.4	16	25	–
15-17	750	1.2	1.7	19	30	–
Girls:						
under 1	450	0.3	0.4	5	20	7.5
1	300	0.4	0.6	7	20	10
2	300	0.5	0.7	8	20	10
3-4	300	0.6	0.8	9	20	10
5-6	300	0.7	0.9	10	20	–
7-8	400	0.8	1.0	11	20	–
9-11	575	0.8	1.2	14	25	–
12-14	725	0.9	1.4	16	25	–
15-17	750	0.9	1.7	19	30	–
Men:						
18-34	750	1.2	1.6	18	30	–
35-64	750	1.1	1.6	18	30	–
65-74	750	1.0	1.6	18	30	–
over 75	750	0.9	1.6	18	30	–
Women:						
18-54	750	0.9	1.3	15	30	–
55-74	750	0.8	1.3	15	30	–
over 75	750	0.7	1.3	15	30	–
pregnant	750	1.0	1.6	18	60	–
lactating	1,200	1.1	1.8	21	60	–

Although recommended intakes are given for vitamin D for infants only, adults who do not get adequate sunlight may require oral vitamin D as this vitamin is produced in the skin by the action of sunlight.

The recommended intake of folic acid is 300 micrograms for all groups.

Essential minerals

Only three minerals (calcium, iron and iodine) have government approved levels. Others are an average based on current opinion.

Calcium	Children 600 mgm; adolescents 700 mgm; adults 500 mgm; in pregnancy and lactation 1200 mgm
Iron	children 6-10 mgm; adolescents and women up to 54 12 mgm; men and elderly women 10 mgm; in pregnancy and lactation 14 mgm
Iodine	150 micrograms
Potassium	(average) 2.54 grams
Magnesium	approx. 400 mgm
Zinc	15-20 mgm

Trace elements

Copper	2 mgm
Manganese	2.5-5.0 mgm
Cobalt	1 microgram
Molybdenum	500 micrograms
Selenium	200 micrograms
Chromium	50-200 mgm
Fluoride	depends on the level of fluoride in the drinking water; approx. 0.5-1.0 mgm

The remaining trace elements, tin, vanadium, silicon, nickel, boron and arsenic, are present in the body, and animals appear to need them. However no function had been discovered in humans, and it is impossible to demonstrate the effects of deficiency as removal from the diet is not an option. They may be significant in disease, as, for example, boron appears to be very low in patients with rheumatoid arthritis. However, they can be toxic in high levels – arsenic is well recognized as a poison!

The function of vitamins and minerals

Vitamin A

This is a fat soluble vitamin, chemical name retinol. It is present only in foods of animal origin, hence deficiency might result from a vegan diet. However, beta-carotene, which is present in vegetables and particularly in carrots, can be converted in the body to vitamin A. The main food sources are fish liver oil, liver, dairy products and eggs.

Primary functions of vitamin A are in sight (particularly night vision), the function of the skin and mucous membranes and in growth. The content of vitamin A in foods is often indicated in international units: 1 microgram vitamin A = 3.3 IU. Daily supplements should not exceed 2,250 micrograms. As it is fat soluble excess intake is possible and this causes dry skin, headaches, nausea and loss of appetite.

Symptoms of deficiency are night blindness, poor hair, dry painful eyes and inflamed mucous membranes.

Vitamin B
There are a number of vitamins in the B group, not all of which appear to play a part in human health.

Vitamin B1
This is commonly known, and labelled, as thiamin. The foods with the highest levels of thiamin are yeast and yeast extract, but significant amounts are also present particularly in brown rice and wheatgerm. Thiamin is an unstable chemical, and is affected by cooking. The function of thiamin is to act as an enzyme, converting glucose into energy.

Deficiency in the West is uncommon, but there is an increased risk during pregnancy and lactation, in those on very low calorie diets and in alcoholics. The symptoms of deficiency are tiredness, muscle weakness, digestive upsets, depression and poor memory. The end result of deficiency is the disease beri-beri, common in third world countries in times of famine.

High doses of thiamin have been used in the treatment of alcoholism, neuralgia and neuritis. High intake does not have any known adverse effects.

Vitamin B2
The chemical name is riboflavin. It has a strong yellow colour, and since the artificial colours, mainly the azo dyes, have fallen from favour, riboflavin is often used as an food colouring agent. In addition to intake in this form in the diet, vitamin B2 is particularly high in yeast and yeast extract, liver, eggs, cheese, wheat bran and meat. Riboflavin is also unstable, and is destroyed by light and in alkaline solutions.

The absorption of riboflavin is affected by alcohol, smoking and the contraceptive pill, and deficiency within these groups is therefore more likely. As it is water soluble, it is safe to take in high dose, the only adverse effect being deep yellow coloured urine.

Vitamin B3

Chemically known as niacin and nicotinic acid. As with many of the B vitamins, again present in high levels in yeast and yeast products, but also high in nuts, wheat bran, liver, meats and oily fish.

Niacin functions as an enzyme, within the cell, and also produces energy from food products. Deficiency is enhanced by alcohol, and in early stages causes diarrhoea, dermatitis, insomnia and irritability. In extreme deficiency, the disease pellegra develops with, in addition, nausea, vomiting, and inflammation of the digestive tract resulting. Excess intake may be harmful, causing flushes and palpitations, and high doses should be avoided during pregnancy. Daily intake should be a minimum of 19 mgm.

Vitamin B4

Chemically this is adenine, at one time thought to be a vitamin, but it is a constituent of DNA and not an essential dietary item.

Vitamin B5

The chemical name for this vitamin is pantothenic acid. Because it is manufactured by bacteria in the intestine, daily intake levels are difficult to assess. However, this also means that the possibility of deficiency will be enhanced by taking antibiotics, as these produce a dysbiosis, destroying the vitamin B5 producing bacteria.

Again, the main food sources are yeast, wheat, liver and nuts. The recommended daily intake is at least 10 mgm, despite the factors mentioned above. There are no reports of symptoms from excess dosage.

Deficiency symptoms are predominantly aching feet with digestive disturbance and abdominal pain. In extreme cases neurological problems develop with depression, insomnia and psychotic symptoms.

Vitamin B6

A water soluble vitamin, known chemically as pyridoxine. Present in the same foods as previously mentioned B vitamins, but significant amounts also appear in bananas and oats. Pyridoxine is commonly taken as a supplement for premenstrual symptoms, as deficiency symptoms are very similar and absorption is reduced by taking the contraceptive pill. However, other drugs, as well as tobacco and alcohol may cause deficiency.

At least 2 mgm per day is required, but supplementation up to 50 mgm a day may be used safely (except in pregnancy), as adverse effects of overdose have only been reported in doses of over 200 mgm a day. These effects are unstable gait and numbness of the hands and feet.

Symptoms of deficiency are cracked lips, depression, breast discomfort, irritability, swollen abdomen and ankles.

Vitamins B7, B8 and B9

These chemicals act as growth factors for bacteria, but have no known function in humans.

Vitamin B10

Not known as essential to humans. Essential for chicks.

Vitamin B12

A water soluble vitamin called cobalamin (or cyano-/hydroxo-cobalamin). This vitamin is almost completely confined to food products of animal origin, and a vegan diet therefore can easily cause deficiency. This results in a sore, smooth tongue, nerve degeneration and symptoms of anaemia. The latter occurs because vitamin B12 is essential for the production of haemoglobin. Vitamin B12 is unusual, because a specific chemical which is produced in the stomach and known as intrinsic factor is needed for its absorption, and when this chemical is not produced pernicious anaemia develops. If this happens the patient has to have occasional injections of vitamin B12 for life.

This vitamin has been used to treat conditions other than anaemia, such as fatigue, mental confusion and poor memory. In addition it was popular until recently to give injections of vitamin B12 as a 'tonic'. The reason it has this effect, if any, is unknown.

Vitamin B13

Chemically this is orotic acid, and it is not now regarded as a vitamin as it is produced within the body. It is also present in foods such as root vegetables. Vitamin B13 has been used, with claims of success, to treat multiple sclerosis (by injection), and chronic hepatitis.

Vitamin Bc

This is more commonly known by its chemical name, folic acid, but it is regarded as one of the B group of vitamins. Present in yeast, wheat, soya, nuts and liver. The possibility of deficiency is enhanced by pregnancy, as well as by drugs and the contraceptive pill. Supplementation during pregnancy is therefore routine in the UK.

Daily needs are 400 micrograms, though higher supplementation is safe, as toxic effects have only been reported in doses of more than 15 milligrams a day or more than thirty-five times the recommended daily dose.

In pregnancy, deficiency results in a typical anaemia, as well as a higher incidence of complications such as toxaemia and premature birth. At other stages of life psychological symptoms occur, with sleeplessness, poor memory and confusion.

Vitamin C

Chemically vitamin C is L-ascorbic acid, and it is water soluble. The main food sources are vegetables and fruits, especially berries. It has a large number of functions in the body, acting as an antioxidant, providing resistance to infection, and maintaining healthy connective tissue, bones and teeth. In addition to dietary lack, there are a number of conditions which predispose to deficiency states. These are stress, infections, injury, high physical activity, old age, diabetes and ingestion of alcohol and a number of drugs.

Although the recommended dose is only in the region of 100 milligrams a day, deficient intake is fairly common in a Western refined diet, particularly for the elderly and those living in institutions, where fresh fruit and vegetables, the main sources, are not readily available.

Scurvy is the disease caused by long-term poor intake, which shows as bleeding gums, easy bruising and joint pains. A low intake which is at a level below that required, but not low enough to cause scurvy, may result in reduced resistance to infection and generalized fatigue. To maintain optimum health an intake of 2 to 3 grams per day is probably required.

As previously mentioned, very high doses, of up to 50 grams, are used by some practitioners to treat chronic infection. If this amount was taken orally diarrhoea would result, which would reduce absorption, and it therefore has to be given by a slow drip directly into the bloodstream.

Vitamin D

The chemical name for vitamin D is cholecalciferol, and it is indicated in international units (1 microgram vitamin D = 40 IU).

Vitamin D is found in liver, oily fish, milk products and egg yolk, as well as being produced in the skin by the action of sunlight. Supplementation, if any, should be largely confined to those who are dark skinned, as they tend to make less vitamin D than fair skinned individuals, and during winter.

Vitamin D is essential for the absorption of calcium and phosphorus, and deficiency therefore affects bone growth and development. In children lack of vitamin D causes rickets, and in adults osteomalacia. Rickets, in the UK, occurs almost exclusively in dark skinned people, resulting in bow legs and knock-knee development of the legs. Osteomalacia in adults (usually the elderly) causes softening of the bones due to lack of calcium.

Vitamin D is the most toxic of all the vitamins, with nausea and vomiting as signs of overdose. Not more than 10 micrograms a day should be taken as supplementation, even in those groups at risk.

Vitamin E

This is a fat soluble vitamin, widely present in the diet, especially in vegetable oils. On supplements it is often shown by its chemical name, tocopherol. Recently it has become popular to take vitamin E, as it is said to slow down the ageing process and to stimulate sexual activity, but high levels of intake are dangerous. Its popularity results from the known functions of vitamin E in preventing thrombosis and arteriosclerosis. This is also why it is used in commercial creams to be applied to wrinkles and stretch marks.

A minimum of 30 milligrams per day is needed, but at least half of this can be gained from even poor diets, so no higher supplementation than 15 milligrams per day is recommended.

Vitamin K

The only known function of this vitamin, also known as phytomenadione, is in blood clotting. It is produced by bacteria in the intestine, and deficiency is therefore almost unknown, except in the newborn where it can cause excessive bleeding from the umbilical stump. One report has also suggested that pregnant women might be deficient. It is also found in green vegetables, kelp, liver, potatoes, eggs and wheat germ.

Daily requirements are unknown, and there are no reports of effects of excess intake.

Calcium

The bones and teeth contain 90% of body calcium, the remainder being predominantly in the blood. In addition to being a basic essential for these tissues, calcium is vital to the conduction of nerve impulses and the contraction of muscles, including the heart. Despite the widely held belief that milk is the major source of calcium in the diet, other foods, particularly nuts, canned fish and white flour (which is fortified with calcium) have higher levels. In addition, some authorities believe that calcium in milk is highly bound and not readily available. Of all the calcium intake in the diet only 20-30% is absorbed, although in deficient states this percentage becomes higher.

Daily requirements are between 400 and 1000 mgm, and excessive intake is virtually impossible unless high doses of vitamin D are also taken, as the body will reject the excess.

Deficiency causes rickets in children, with deformation of bones, and osteomalacia in adults, producing bone pain, but both these conditions are more commonly due to decrease in vitamin D production.

Magnesium

The body contains approximately 25 grams of magnesium, half of this within the bones. Around 400 mgm per day is the necessary intake, and much of this in hard water areas will be obtained from drinking water. Other dietary sources are soya, nuts, wheat and flour. There is some evidence that magnesium deficiency may be related to heart disease, as this condition is more prevalent in soft water areas and heart muscle of sufferers shows a lower magnesium level.

Deficiency is aggravated by infections, overuse of laxatives, poor diet, high milk intake and kidney disease. A number of drugs interfere with absorption, notably antibiotics, the contraceptive pill and diuretics.

A recent report showed that patients with chronic fatigue syndrome were deficient in magnesium, possibly through poor absorption. Magnesium deficiency, as with zinc, may be very common due to lower levels of magnesium in foods in recent decades, and some recommend a daily intake of 800 milligrams.

Potassium
This is one of the most prevalent minerals in the body, with about 140 grams present in the average adult. Potassium is contained in a wide range of foods, but the actual amount varies according to processing. The main sources are raw salad vegetables and fruit, and as these are often not major food items for the elderly, potassium deficiency is relatively common in this age group. In addition, diuretic drugs, which promote excretion of fluid, also increase the excretion of potassium, and these drugs are commonly taken by the elderly. Other conditions which make deficiency more likely are intestinal surgery and persistent vomiting or diarrhoea.

The symptoms of deficiency includes vomiting (which only worsens the problem), drowsiness and muscular weakness. Supplements of potassium should be taken by anyone on diuretics and those who have an inadequate diet.

Phosphorus
This chemical, combined with oxygen, is present in all cells. It is so common in foods that deficiency is almost unknown, except in patients with rickets and osteomalacia as the levels of absorption are dependent on sufficient vitamin D.

Sulphur
Again, this element is so common in the diet that effects of too low an intake are unknown. Any diet sufficiently low in sulphur or phosphorus would produce symptoms of deficiency of other vitamins and minerals before their lack produced effects. Sulphur is mainly present in the hair, nails and skin, linking the 'building blocks' of these tissues – the higher the sulphur content, the curlier the hair.

Iron

Supplementary iron, unless it is deficient in the diet, is dangerous as it increases the risk of liver disease. Iron functions mainly as a part of the structure of haemoglobin, the oxygen carrying chemical in the blood, so inadequate intake causes a characteristic anaemia, with typical symptoms of tiredness and pale complexion.

As the main source of dietary iron is meat, deficiency may occur in vegetarians, and supplementation may also be needed if there is excessive bleeding (e.g. heavy periods). In pregnancy the requirements are increased and supplementation is therefore routine. Iron taken by mouth can cause digestive upset. The recommended intake varies according to age and sex.

Zinc

Zinc deficiency is probably very common in people on Western diets. Two studies have shown that this may be as high as 70-80% of the population. This is probably due to two factors – food processing removes up to 80% of the zinc, and due to overproduction the soil in cultivated areas is low in zinc, as is the food grown there. Zinc deficiency is therefore a result of twentieth century life.

Unfortunately the food containing the highest zinc levels, with ten times the amount of other foods, is hardly an everyday item – oysters! The fact that zinc deficiency results in impaired sexual ability and function probably accounts for the reputation oysters have gained as an aphrodisiac.

There is no danger in taking extra zinc, unless this exceeds 100 milligrams a day. The probable daily need is around 25 milligrams, and the best form appears to be zinc citrate.

Copper

Much of the copper in our diets is not contained in the foodstuffs but comes from the processing and transport of food. Copper cooking vessels, water pipes, pesticides in foods, all contribute copper. It seems therefore that copper supplements are probably not needed, as the daily requirement is only 2 milligrams. However, one research study showed that the diet of 75% of Americans *was* below the required copper level – though this did not take into account the copper in drinking water.

Manganese
Deficiency is rare as this is so common in the diet, especially in tea drinking countries – five cups provides all the daily need.

Boron
Until recently boron compounds were used as preservatives in food, but it became clear that intakes in excess of 100 milligrams a day caused toxicity. Boron preservatives are therefore now banned. In some ways this is unfortunate, as there is increasing evidence that boron is an essential trace element, which may be too low in some diets. Boron was, until recently, only thought to be essential to plants.

In countries where soil levels of boron are high, and hence levels in food are high, arthritis only affects a small proportion of the population, and rheumatoid arthritis is virtually unknown. In addition, it has been shown that patients with rheumatoid arthritis have extremely low levels of boron. Perhaps boron supplementation, in a dose of 3-5 mgm a day, may reduce the risk of arthritis.

Cobalt
Cobalt is a constituent of vitamin B12, and dietary deficiency therefore only occurs when the intake of this vitamin is low.

Molybdenum
As with zinc and boron, molybdenum deficiency is associated solely with the consumption of foods from soil which itself is deficient. However, dietary needs are so low that deficiency is rare. The result is dental caries. Excess intake can be harmful in that it has been reported to cause gout.

Selenium
Only in the last few years has it been thought that selenium is an essential trace element. Patients fed by drip which did not contain selenium showed symptoms which were reversed by the addition of selenium. It probably acts by enhancing the effect of other vitamins and minerals, notably vitamin E, and magnesium. Lower levels of these appear to be needed if adequate selenium is taken. As with molybdenum and boron, selenium is found in vegetables and grains; its concentration depends on the amount in the soil.

Excess levels can be dangerous, so supplements should not be more than 200 micrograms a day.

Chromium
Intake of chromium in the diet is usually adequate, though only a very small proportion – less than 10% – is absorbed. It is found in fresh unprocessed foods such as grains, nuts, fruit and brewer's yeast. The main function is the activation of insulin, and deficiency results in symptoms of diabetes – indeed it may be related to the cause of diabetes. Oddly, chromium levels in the body vary according to race – from less than 6 milligrams in the West to over 12 milligrams in the Far East. Whether this is due to diet is not known.

As no effects from overdose have been reported it is probably safe to take up to 200 micrograms daily.

Fluoride
The function of fluoride is not fully known, but it appears to give strength to bones and teeth. The first symptom of low fluoride intake is dental decay, and it is for this reason that fluoride is added to water. Ironically an excess intake may inhibit calcium levels.

As well as intake from drinking water, fluoride occurs in foods, particularly cereals, and the level is high in tea (especially China tea).

Nickel
Although known to be essential in animals and present in minute amounts in human tissues, it is unclear as to whether nickel is an essential mineral. Toxic effects are unknown, but allergy to nickel, not only from skin contact but also from excess intake, appears to be an occasional problem. The main food sources are due to contamination – for example from the metal of cooking utensils.

Silicon
This is an essential component of cartilage and connective tissue, but studies of deficiency and excess have, so far, been confined to animal experiments. When inhaled, silicon dust causes the lung disease silicosis.

Arsenic, tin and vanadium
These elements should be mentioned as there is some evidence that they may be needed in minute amounts. Arsenic is, of course, toxic in anything but the smallest traces. Certainly there is much evidence for their need in animals. These trace

elements are found in the soil and hence absorbed via grains, vegetables and fresh fruit.

Toxic minerals

Three minerals are usually found in the human adult which are not needed, are poisonous at high levels, and are purely the result of 'civilised' modern life. Lead is taken into the body primarily from car exhaust fumes, and from plants grown in contaminated soil such as near main roads. Indeed, lead contamination is now so widespread that there is not one area of the UK where the soil is uncontaminated. Earlier sources of lead poisoning, such as lead containing paint and lead water pipes have now been eliminated, but soil contamination is more worrying as it is insidious, increasing and impossible to reverse.

Cadmium contamination occurs near industrial works such as smelting plants. Some degree of cadmium intake occurs in the majority of the population, and again, in the absence of legislation, appears to be on the increase.

There is considerable debate regarding the origin of mercury found in modern man. It seems probable that this may come from the 'leakage' of mercury from dental amalgams (fillings), though a more well defined source is contaminated fish from areas which discharge mercury compounds such as Japan. Industrial air pollution is another possible source.

Testing for vitamin and mineral deficiency

Unfortunately it is far from easy to assess the levels of vitamins and minerals in a person. Some are in such minute amounts that they are untraceable by usual methods, and others only show their absence by their effects – such as pernicious anaemia. Another complicating factor is that the level in the blood may be artificially high if a food containing high levels has been recently eaten.

Often each substance, particularly the minerals, is best shown by its level in a particular tissue. The level of zinc in the sweat, for example, appears to be the best indicator for overall zinc level, whereas for magnesium the ideal indicator seems to be the level inside red blood cells. As a screening method for mineral status the best test is probably a hair analysis, as this reflects the state of the mineral level over several months. Unfortunately even this has problems, as deficiencies may affect hair growth and hence the outcome.

An 'ideal' supplement for health

Although modification according to lifestyle, drug intake and age may be needed, the following supplementation could be taken by a healthy adult. Suggested levels are safe for possibly toxic items.

Vitamin A	2,000 micrograms
Vitamin B1	1.5 milligrams
Vitamin B2	1.5 milligrams
Vitamin B6	20 milligrams
Vitamin B12	3 micrograms
Folic Acid	400 micrograms
Vitamin C	1000 milligrams
Vitamin E	15 milligrams
Magnesium	200 milligrams
Zinc	25 milligrams

Other essential items should be present in adequate amounts in the diet.

PART III

Specific diseases associated with allergy and factors underlying multiple allergies

CHAPTER 12

Electromagnetism and its effect on health

Most family doctors know that there are areas in their practice where certain diseases seem particularly common. Sometimes the area may be very small, in that one street may appear to have a high incidence of a particular illness. Even one house may be successively occupied by a person who develops cancer whilst living there – so-called 'cancer houses'. Architects now recognize the problem of the 'sick building syndrome' where illness seems more common – but its cause is unknown. Perhaps the reason for both these phenomena is the pollution which has only appeared this century and has not left a corner of the planet unaffected. A pollution which is particularly worrying as it is both invisible and intangible.

We have, until the last few years, accepted electricity as a boon to our way of life to the extent that we are now highly dependent on a continuous and reliable supply. This acceptance of its value has created an assumption that it is without risk – except by direct contact, as an electrical shock. Unfortunately there are through history many examples of environmental pollution thought, at the time, to be harmless, which have subsequently proved otherwise – the risks from overdosage of X-rays, inhalation of asbestos, and more recently the gas in aerosols causing the 'hole' in the ozone layer are three examples. Possibly electricity, which since its discovery has been assumed to be without danger, is a greater threat than any of these.

Electromagnetic fields

Around any electrical cable or appliance there is an area in which the electricity can be detected by sensitive instruments.

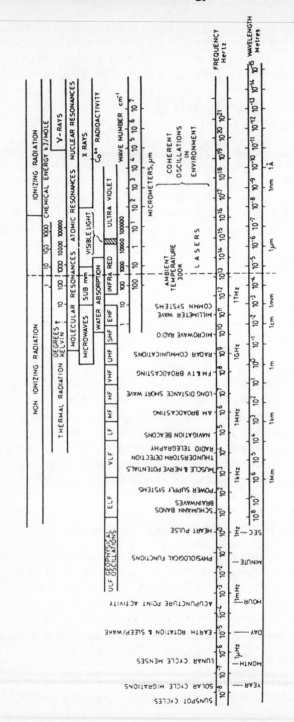

The electromagnetic spectrum.

As well as this electrical field or area there is also a magnetic field, similar to the magnetic field of the earth. The size of the area affected depends on the voltage and current being carried; thus for domestic appliances at 240 volts with a relatively low current it will only be a matter of inches, but for an overhead power cable, carrying possibly 400,000 volts it may be several tens or hundreds of yards.

Until the eighteenth century, when electricity was discovered, the only electromagnetic radiation to which humans were exposed was caused by the natural fields from the earth itself and small amounts from sources in space. Since then, human exposure has increased ten thousand times, most of that increase being in the last fifty years with the widespread development of radio, radar, television and electrical transmission. There is now nowhere on earth unaffected by this electromagnetic pollution.

Fields from the transmission of electricity are only a small part of the range of electromagnetic fields, which includes radio and television transmission, microwaves, nuclear radiation and even visible light. The variable factor is the frequency, from below 300 cycles per second (extremely low frequencies – ELF), to gamma rays at millions of cycles per second. The higher frequencies are known as ionising radiation as they have the ability to split an electron from the atom, and these are known to be harmful to health.

The non-ionising frequencies are the ones that currently cause concern. Microwaves in sufficient dosage can produce heating of the body and be harmful (hence the screening around microwave cookers). What is not clear is whether doses which do not have a heating effect are also harmful.

The electricity transmission system

Prior to the development of the national grid electricity in the UK was generated by small local stations and distributed to the immediate area. Because the distances involved were short, it was possible to use a low voltage. When the national grid was set up, connecting all electricity stations, it became necessary to carry supplies over hundreds of miles, and with these distances if a low voltage was used the loss in transit would be considerable. Electricity is therefore now carried at a maximum voltage of 400,000 volts, which is reduced at sub-stations on the edge of towns and cities to 125,000 volts, and eventually by local sub-stations to the domestic voltage. For technical reasons the national grid was also standardized to operate using an alternating current in which the flow oscillates back and forth instead of using a continuous forward flow. In this country the frequency, or rate of oscillation, was set at fifty times per second. This therefore produces an electromagnetic field of 50 cycles per second.

Although the maximum voltage supposedly carried in the system is 400,000 volts, there can be moments, lasting fractions of a second, when several million volts may be carried. This is due to switching in and out of various sections of the grid. Obviously such a large increase, even though very brief, dramatically increases the power and range of the electromagnetic field. It may be that these brief but very high exposures are relevant to health, in the same way that a low powered electric shock may be no more than unpleasant, but a high voltage shock, even if very brief, can be fatal.

Electromagnetic toxicity

Concern over the problem – or potential problem – varies considerably from one country to another. The Russians were the first to identify a possible risk when they noticed that workers who in their job were exposed to fields had a higher incidence of illness. This led to them adopting limits for exposure to electromagnetic fields, which are the strictest in the world. A Russian worker is limited to three hours per day exposure to fields which in this country can be encountered in homes under high voltage cables. In America there is now a 'right of way' around transmission cables within which domestic buildings cannot be erected. In the UK no such legislation exists – the decision rests with the local planning authority. There *are* recommended limits for exposure, but these are one thousand times higher than that considered safe in the most cautious countries.

Not only is the USSR the most cautious regarding exposure of its citizens to electromagnetic fields, but it is possibly the most knowledgeable about the use of such fields in defence and surveillance. In 1977 it was revealed that Russia had been irradiating the American embassy in Moscow with microwaves since 1953 in an attempt to eavesdrop on internal communications. Several members of the embassy staff have since claimed that this irradiation had adverse effects on their health, and the three ambassadors serving in Moscow during that time have since died of cancer. In recent years an electromagnetic beam of very, very low frequency (about 10 cycles per second – hence known to the military as the 'woodpecker') has been detected between Russia and America. Which country is producing it, and its purpose, is a closely guarded secret.

Concern in the UK about the possible health effects from overhead transmission lines started in 1975, when a group of residents at a small village in Dorset, Fishpond Bottom, complained to the Central Electricity Generating Board. They claimed that the 400,000 volt line, passing directly over their houses, was responsible for a variety of ailments including depression, insomnia, headaches and even cancer. Their allegations were entirely rejected by the CEGB, and this rejection was supported by the Department of the Environment. Unfortunately shortly *after* this enquiry two important studies were revealed. The first, from the USA indicated an increase in leukaemia in children who were exposed to magnetic fields from wiring near their homes. The second showed that the magnetic field in the homes of people who had committed suicide was higher than in other homes.

Other studies followed; an investigation into the cause of death in workers who were exposed to electromagnetic fields through their occupation showed that there was an increase of 25% in leukaemia compared to the general population. Recently a comparison of chronic ill health in the occupants of houses under a power line compared to a similar group with no power line demonstrated an increase in recurrent headaches and depression. In this investigation it was found that the condition was also related to proximity to the line – so perhaps the condition caused is dependent on the strength of the field.

Effects from domestic supply
Because of the relatively low voltage and low current through the wiring of houses the range of any significant field is probably only inches. Only by being close to an appliance or to wires carrying a current for several hours could one be exposed to sufficient radiation – and even this remains controversial. One study from the USA suggests that women sleeping under electric blankets or on heated water beds (which carry a current all night) have an increased risk of miscarriage. Until the issue is clearer it is probably advisable to avoid such devices

137

and not to sleep near a cable which is connected to an appliance switched on most of the time (such as a refrigerator).

A special case

Over a period of two years the occupants of a small bungalow in Gloucestershire experienced a series of domestic disasters which appeared unconnected and inexplicable. Through sudden electrical failure they lost more than fifteen domestic appliances, experienced over twenty minor fires due to electrical cables, suffered from headaches and depression, and noticed that some domestic animals had died without explanation. In addition to the electrical system being affected, there were plumbing leaks due to the loosening of joints or the implosion of pipes.

Careful plotting of the disasters showed that they occurred in a corridor some eight feet wide through the building, and extension of this line terminated at one end at a dish communications aerial, and at the other at GCHQ at Cheltenham. Not surprisingly an association was denied by the authorities, but a team of experts decided that the only possible explanation was interference with the electrical supply by high electromagnetic frequencies (such as beamed radio transmission). Curiously, but perhaps not coincidentally, all the effects stopped after the problem was highlighted on a television programme.

US inquiry

Because of the public concern such findings caused, an inquiry was ordered in 1979 into the proposal for the erection of a 765,000 volt line from the Canadian border to New York. Although the proposal was eventually approved, two important conditions were imposed at the inquiry. The first demanded that a 350 foot wide corridor, or right of way, should be established around the line, within which no residence would be permitted. The second required that a research programme, at a cost of five million dollars and largely funded by the power authorities, should take place into the health effects of transmission lines. This condition resulted in the New York State Power Lines Project, which finally presented its report in July 1987.

The report is precise, detailed, and consequently a lengthy document. It deals not only with the results of the various projects, but also with the physics of electromagnetic fields, particularly those surrounding power lines. Details of the variety of projects are given, together with a summary of the results.

The studies were basically in four areas: reproduction and development, cancer, cell biology, and neurobiology and behaviour. Effects were accepted in two of these (cancer and behaviour), though some studies supported effects in the other two.

Power lines, as previously mentioned, produce both electric and magnetic fields, and it is concluded in the report that the latter are of more importance when considering possible health hazards. It states: 'Magnetic field effects were found in a number of studies in this program ... The epidemiological studies raise the possibility that magnetic flux density one-thousandth of those shown to have effects in laboratory studies may be a health concern.'

In the studies on animal behaviour it was shown that whilst fields do not directly appear to affect adult learning, interaction between the earth's magnetic field and power line fields can influence behaviour, but that this is temporary and only occurs during exposure. On the other hand, 'prenatal exposure to these fields produces more or less permanent changes in response activity'.

The conclusions regarding cancer, particularly leukaemia in children are of more concern. Regarding one of the studies, it states that: 'Even though the Savitz study ... has certain limitations, it indicates an excess risk for childhood cancer, in particular leukaemias, associated with high current wiring configuration near the home.' Furthermore, they stated that if the association suggested by this study is true then the leukaemia rate for children exposed to fields would be *double* that of an unexposed group, and that '10-15% of all childhood cancer cases are attributable to magnetic fields'.

Despite this report the CEGB has persisted in denying the possibility of any effects. They *have* carried out research, but usually on small numbers or on short term exposure, not the effects on people in their homes. Early in 1988 they announced a further research project at a cost of £500,000, but details are not yet forthcoming. Curiously the announcement of this project was made a few days before a television documentary highlighting the research undertaken abroad.

It would be wrong to give the impression that *all* electromagnetic fields are detrimental. Indeed, it has been convincingly shown that a magnetic field at a particular frequency applied across a fractured bone increases the rate of healing. It may well be shown that particular frequencies and strengths are preventative to ill health – there is a greater amount not known about the problem than known at present.

Other factors may be important. Local geology may be significant in producing a higher than average magnetic field from the earth, which in turn may resonate, interfere with or amplify any man-made fields. It seems at present that areas which are low lying and have water near the surface could be particularly important, though whether this is because the earth's field is greater, or whether, because of ground conditions, cables are carried overhead, is not clear.

On the balance of evidence it is becoming apparent that electromagnetic fields *do* have an effect on health, but this is probably only one factor of many – in the same way as smoking is one factor in the development of lung cancer. Understanding its relative importance depends on further research. In the meantime we should perhaps act on the side of caution and avoid any unnecessary exposure – preferably by legislation.

Allergy – or sensitivity – to electromagnetic fields

Quite apart from the toxic effects of exposure, as discussed so far, there remains the problem that certain individuals may react to levels of exposure far lower than those which would affect most people. This is directly comparable to the situation with chemical exposure, where high levels will have adverse effects on everyone, whereas some people react to a much lower dose.

In the same way in which a sensitivity to a chemical, pollen or other environmental pollutant develops, the sensitivity to electromagnetic fields arises due to exposure, usually at continuous or high levels, to particular frequencies. In later life the patient may then develop symptoms when exposed at much lower levels.

CASE HISTORY

A 35 year old housewife noticed that she developed symptoms following a move to a new house. These consisted of extreme fatigue, headaches and dizzy spells. She also realized that when away from the house for more than a few days there was considerable improvement in her symptoms. Testing showed that symptoms developed at the precise frequency used for the radar directing aircraft on their landing path, and an examination of a map showed that her new home was on the flight path for a major airport – albeit at several tens of miles distant. She then mentioned that as a child she had lived very near an airport due to her father's job. It would appear that her childhood exposure had sensitized her to low levels of exposure encountered in later life.

Sensitivity to electromagnetic fields may be extreme and dramatic. One patient developed epileptic fits when in the region of high voltage overhead power lines, even though unaware of their presence. Another, a six year old, had dramatic changes in her behaviour when a local dish transmitting aerial was directed towards her home. Of all sensitivities, these examples may seem far-fetched, but increasingly it appears to be a real problem in our electro-polluted world.

Testing for electromagnetic sensitivity

One would imagine that it would be relatively easy to test patients to see if they are reacting to electromagnetic fields simply by exposing them. But the situation is much more complex, as there is nowhere where the exposure is unaffected by other sources. It is therefore of paramount importance to provide a 'clean' electromagnetic room in which to test patients. The only way in which this can be provided is by screening a room, all round, with wire mesh and sheet aluminium. In this room are placed oscillators, which produce fields at known frequencies, to which the patient can be exposed. At present there are only three such testing facilities in the world.

If symptoms appear to occur in a patient, at definite frequencies, then it is usually possible to confirm this by returning to those frequencies, unknown to the patient, to see if symptoms once again happen. In this way it is possible, though time consuming, to identify patients with genuine electromagnetic sensitivity.

Management of electromagnetically sensitive patients

If a patient's sensitivity is extreme, it may be that the only possible answer is for them to avoid exposure. This may involve a move of house or job, if the source can be identified.

In less extreme cases desensitization may be possible. When testing patients, not only are frequencies found which cause symptoms, other frequencies are discovered which improve symptoms. This is directly comparable to the 'switch-off' dilution with other sensitivities. It is possible to 'imprint' this frequency into water, which the patients then take as 'medicine' in order to maintain their exposure to their switch-off frequency. It appears that the molecules of water will vibrate at the frequency to which they have been exposed, and will maintain this vibrational quality thus also radiating that frequency, for about two weeks. This ties in with patients' observations that their 'medicine' loses its 'power' after two weeks.

Of all areas of allergy and environmental medicine, electromagnetic sensitivity remains the most open to criticism, but at the same time the most exciting. Worldwide electromagnetic pollution has been unrecognized as a potential health problem, possibly because it has been with us a relatively short time. In another fifty years we may realise that it is a factor in the causation of ill health to the same extent as other environmental pollutants.

CHAPTER 13

Toxicity

There can be no doubt that toxicity due to the bewildering array of poisons which we breathe in, eat and rub on our skins, is a major underlying cause of food, chemical and airborne sensitivity. Toxicity is particularly likely to trigger allergic disease such as asthma, or ulcerative colitis, in those already genetically predisposed because of an allergic family history. In this chapter we will outline the theory of toxicity, as viewed from a naturopathic point of view. The naturopathic description of toxicity does sound eminently sensible and coherent, even though it cannot claim to be scientifically proven and it also provides a useful framework on which to hang the hat of treatment for the clearance of toxins from the body. Conventional medical research is beginning to publish evidence that substantiates many of the ideas that we are going to discuss here and as a consequence we believe the concept and treatment of toxicity will become increasingly important.

Natural defences

So far as the naturopaths are concerned, illness is the end result of a battle between toxins and the body's natural defences. The most important part of the body's defences lies in the immune system. Many of the medications used in complementary medicine, particularly combinations of herbal and homoeopathic remedies known as complex homoeopathy, stimulate the immune system in order to facilitate the body's immune competence.

Naturopaths believe that the autonomic nervous system (the part of the nervous system controlling unconscious internal body functions such as heart rate, intestinal muscle contraction, etc.) has a major part to play in balancing the body's natural defences between activity (stimulated by the sympathetic division of the autonomic nervous system) and quies-

cence (encouraged by the parasympathetic division of the autonomic nervous system). There is increasing evidence from the
basic medical sciences that this may well be so. Also many of
the natural therapies such as acupuncture and osteopathy
work through the autonomic nervous system and therefore can
be expected to improve the body's natural defences.

The second arm of the body's defences lies in its methods of
getting rid of toxins via three main routes of excretion: the
colon, the kidneys and the skin. Methods of encouraging stimulation via these routes using intestinal stimulants, diuretics
(which increase urine flow) and diaphoretics (substances that
increase sweating) are the cornerstone of naturopathic and
herbal practice. A fundamental feature of complex
homoeopathic therapy embodies these principles by including
herbal preparations in complex homoeopathic mixtures to encourage toxin elimination.

The third arm of our natural defences is the lymphatic
system. This consists of a vast network of tiny capillaries which
permeate all the connective tissues of the body. The lymphatics
drain tissue fluid away together with toxins into large aggrega-
tions of lymphatic tissue known as lymph nodes. The toxins
carried by the lymph are largely excreted in the intestine via
the so-called Peyer's patches of lymphatic tissue situated just
below the internal lining of the small intestine. The lymph
system acts like an internal connective tissue cleansing system. Anything which impedes its flow or overwhelms it with
toxins will soon give rise to a local accumulation of toxins,
depending on where the problem is. Also a slight rise in
pressure inside the small intestine may prejudice the fine
balance which allows the lymphatics to discharge into the
intestine via the Peyer's patches.

Many complex homoeopathic medicaments contain effective
lymphatic stimulants; this is one of the important mechanisms
contributing to the effectiveness of this form of therapy. Exercise also has the effect of improving lymphatic flow, therefore
many people with food sensitivities or indeed any chronic
illness may feel improved following exercise. This helps toxin
excretion, not only through the lymphatic system, but clearly it
also increases sweating which is another means of discharging
toxins. Habitual constipation can be a major problem as it
predisposes to toxins remaining in the lymphatic system. We
have a lot to learn from the Victorian obsession with 'bowels' as

unfortunately much of modern medicine has lost sight of these simple facts.

Toxins

Toxins are defined as any poisonous substance present in the body. The list below gives the most common ones, but they are not placed in any order of toxicity. Some are clearly more poisonous than others and this depends on many factors beside the toxicity of the substance itself, such as the amount present and the state or health of the tissues. As a rule, toxins in chronic disease are not acutely poisonous but produce their effects by being present in the tissues in small amounts and continually accumulating there if exposure is continued over a long period of time. Unfortunately the body tends to store toxins most commonly in the fat cells and in various organs. Some toxins have a preference for particular organs such as the liver or the nervous system. What then happens is that enzymes, particularly in the liver, become overwhelmed by the sheer volume of poisonous substance. This is probably why nutritional therapy can be so effective in multiple sensitivity (see Chapter 11), as many minerals, particularly magnesium and zinc, are important components of a vast range of enzymes in the body.

Common toxins include:
Industrial chemicals.
Pesticides, weedkillers and insecticides.
Food additives.
Bacteria – often the material from the dead bodies of bacteria (which is made of protein) acts as the toxin. Live bacteria themselves are rarely toxic, but can produce chemicals which, in turn, are well recognized poisons. These chemicals, such as streptolysin produced by dividing streptococci bacteria, are usually clinically manifest during acute illness such as scarlet fever. Toxins in the present sense are usually far less poisonous than substances such as streptolysin.
Viruses – as in bacterial toxins this usually refers to parts of the dead viral body.
Conventional medical drugs – especially antibiotics and mood changing drugs such as antidepressants and anti-anxiety drugs such as valium.

Hydrocarbon based chemicals.

Heavy metals – such as lead and mercury. The most common source of mercury toxicity is from dental amalgam (the material out of which most dental fillings are made).

Phases of toxicity

The first phase, called the humoral phase, is one in which the toxins are present in the extracellular fluid which bathes all the cells in our body. Towards the end of this phase they are beginning to move into the cells. This phase is characterized by attempts by the body to excrete these toxins, via the colon, urinary tract and the skin.

The second phase, known as the cellular degeneration phase, starts with the toxins in the cells, progresses with increasing cellular degeneration and ends with cancer. In the present context cancer is viewed as the extreme end of the degenerative process, implying an assumed toxic cause of cancer. During the second phase any attempts by the body to excrete toxins have no effect as the important toxins are locked away inside the cells.

Each phase is subdivided into three sub-phases, shown in the following table. Underneath each phase are examples from particular diseases which clarify the concept of toxin deposition and degeneration.

As shown on the chart, progression of disease to the humoral excretion phase is the natural history of improving your health. Conversely progression to the neoplastic phase is the natural history of chronic disease. Simple measures to aid toxin excretion will help most situations in the humoral phase. Homoeopathic dilutions of toxins are essential in the cellular degeneration phase. It is interesting to note that there is a large volume of well conducted research within homoeopathy, which shows quite clearly that non-material dilutions of toxins, such as lead, arsenic or copper, are able to get the body to excrete these poisons. Some of this work has been carried out on plants, much of it is very elegant and most convincing. We are of the opinion that the use of nosodes (homoeopathic dilutions of toxins), are an essential part of detoxification.

HUMORAL PHASE			CELLULAR DEGENERATION PHASE		
Excretion phase	Reaction phase	Deposition phase	Impregnation phase	Degeneration phase	Neoplastic (cancerous) phase
Characterized by the body attempting to get rid of toxins via faeces, urine, catarrh, menstrual bleeding, discharges from infected wounds, etc.	Characterized by inflammatory reactions e.g. ezcema, enteritis, pharyngitis, tonsillitis, appendicitis, etc.	Characterized by more or less permanent cellular change due to toxin deposition, e.g. gout, benign tumours, cysts, rheumatism, etc.	Characterized by toxins being present in the cell such as liver damage (cirrhosis), various lung diseases, e.g. pneumoconiosis (due to long term exposure to coal dust) or asbestosis (due to exposure to asbestos).	Characterized by cellular degeneration due to long standing presence of toxins in the cells e.g. osteoarthritis, myocardial infarction (heart attack), emphysema.	Characterized by malignant change and the development of cancer in the tissues affected by the toxins.

There is a very important barrier between the two phases which is sometimes known as the biological sesura. Once any disease is over this barrier it is much more difficult to treat, as organic cell damage is present. Therefore the further the progression to the right the more difficult it is to institute effective therapy. This is not so much because the toxins cannot be removed from the cells, but more because the body becomes increasingly debilitated the more it moves to the right. This is characterized by depletion of increasing numbers of essential enzymes, minerals and vitamins. The emerging science of nutritional medicine has something valuable to offer here by restoking the body's essential supplies of these substances. Often the only effective way of enabling an exhausted debilitated patient to respond to causally directed therapy is to prescribe intensive nutritional medical therapy specifically aimed at the deficiencies found (see Chapter 11). This sort of therapy may have to be continued for many months before a useful improvement occurs.

Any therapy which suppresses any of the phases illustrated in the table will encourage toxins to move into the cell, and therefore increase the risk of chronic degenerative illness or cancer. Causal treatment is therefore based on helping the cells to excrete the toxins out into the extracellular fluid which bathes the cells, and from there to expel them from the body.

CASE HISTORY

Jane is aged 43. She began to notice a slow steady decline in her general health, with no specific symptoms, when she moved to a country village just outside Southampton. She also noticed that many pets in the area seemed to become ill when their owners moved there. Her symptoms were very non-specific, consisting of general lack of energy, muscle aching, and some degree of indigestion and occasional loose bowels. On careful questioning we found that she lived downwind of a large strawberry farm, and her symptoms were always worse in the spring and summer when the strawberry farmer liberally sprayed his strawberry crop with pesticides, weedkillers and herbicides. Jane only began to improve when we gave her homoeopathic nosodes (homoeopathic dilutions of toxins), made from weedkillers and pesticides. This was accompanied by a liver and kidney remedy in order to help her excrete these toxins out of the body. Initially there was some degree of aggravation in her symptoms as the toxins began to be excreted. Gradually she became better and better, and she was able to regain 70% of her previous level of health. She was only able to completely regain her health on moving away from the area.

The role of bacteria

Bacteria are popularly regarded as being universally harmful, yet they are essential to life (see Chapter 15). It is interesting to note that most bacteria found in inflamed tissues are also found performing essential functions in the gall bladder, the intestines or on the skin. The naturopathic view of toxicity suggests that bacteria mop up the toxins present in the extracellular fluid by engulfing and digesting them. In other words, the bacteria perform a useful function and once the poisons have been removed the bacteria will die and disappear. Furthermore, bacterial infection might not have occurred in the first place if poisons had not been present in the tissues. This implies that it is the terrain and not the bacteria which is the most important fact. For example, one common and interesting finding is that cholera bacteria, when taken into the body, do not always cause cholera in all those who ingest them. Only those people who have the necessary toxins present, or whose immune systems are compromised in some way, and are by implication 'under par' as far as their health is concerned, will succumb. Similar findings have been made in other bacterial and viral infections.

Other mechanisms of toxicity, free oxidizing radicals

Oxygen is essential to life and it has an ability to react with many substances, particularly when it is present as a free oxidizing radical (FOR) as in hydrogen peroxide (H_2O_2) as opposed to water (H_2O). Some ecologists are beginning to use hydrogen peroxide medicinally with, in some cases, remarkable results. White blood cells produce peroxides when they attack invading bacteria in the blood or tissues. Therefore giving hydrogen peroxide medicinally is simply strengthening a mechanism which the body is already using.

The levels of FORs have to be kept within certain limits, otherwise they can wreak havoc by causing extensive biochemical damage to the tissues. Smog (air pollution), exhaust fumes, pesticides, insecticides and weedkillers all produce adverse effects on all of us, partly by producing an excess for FORs in the body. Some people respond to this with running eyes and nose, but those who get no such symptoms may well be storing up long-term problems for themselves by FOR exposure. Foods such as coffee are also major sources.

Because FORs are primarily electron donors they are particularly good at splitting double bonds and this is responsible for many of their damaging effects on the body. An important area where double bonds are essential is in DNA (deoxyribonucleic acid), out of which chromosomes are made. DNA consists of two parallel strands of compounds known as nucleotides which are held together by sulphur-sulphur double bonds. The nucleotides themselves also contain double bonds, all of which are vulnerable to damage by the FORs. If DNA becomes disturbed as a result of this mechanism it cannot provide correct information for cell division, resulting in a deterioration in the efficiency of protein manufacture, with the consequent depletion of vital enzyme systems. Also destruction of the DNA may lead to abnormal cells which in some cases may develop into cancer.

All our cells contain, and are surrounded by, complex membrane systems which are made of specialized fats called phosopho-lipids. They are arranged in specific ways due to the electrical forces in their double bonds. These are particularly vulnerable to attack by FORs, which can consequently lead to cellular destruction. Luckily we have antioxidant systems in the body which limit the formation of FORs. These are vitamins A and E (fat soluble vitamins) and vitamin C (water soluble). Unfortunately the average British diet is deficient in all these vitamins, particularly vitamins A and C. Coupled with our increasing exposure to chemicals and air pollution, this means that the health risks of these toxins are multiplied. Clearly a healthy nutritional approach would diminish the risks with a diet high in vegetables (especially raw vegetables as cooking destroys many essential nutrients). Surprisingly enough it is only recently that a major epidemiological study has been published which shows that people who have a diet high in vegetables are less at risk from cancer than those with a lower vegetable intake. Clearly the FORs and the antioxidant vitamins A, E and C could explain this finding.

Conclusion

It is clear that toxicity, which is becoming more common in the civilized world, is a major cause of chronic illness and the major underlying feature of multiple food and chemical sensitivity. Our own conclusion is that the scientific proof of toxicity is a myth and ought to be generally seen as such. It really all depends on the individual as to whether a substance is toxic or not. Somebody who is in a very debilitated state will be much more susceptible to very low levels of toxins than somebody who is in a robust state of health. The safest option for the average person is to take appropriate steps to limit exposure using the various methods suggested in this chapter and maintain optimal nutrition. The sceptic may well regard all of this as unproven, which in a strict scientific sense it is. But unfortunately the chances are that he or she will have succumbed to the toxins long before any of the quality of proven evidence he or she requires is on the horizon!

CHAPTER 14

Candida

Candida, also known as thrush, is a fungus which is usually known for the infection it causes in the vagina in women. The candida organism is normally present in a healthy gut, but it is in a harmless form in which the cells are spherical in form. In patients with candidiasis, the cells change their shape, becoming elongated, attached together and forming a 'cobweb' over the inside of the intestine. This occurs because of suppression of the normally protective bacteria in the gut, and because these candida cells form 'roots' to attach themselves to the intestinal wall. This in turn allows the absorption into the circulation of proteins, thus setting up sensitivities. It is for this reason that candida itself has secondary effects in causing food intolerances.

This problem is commonly present in people with depressed immune systems, and those with post viral syndromes or myalgic encephalomyelitis. It is important to understand that candida is naturally present (in its harmless spherical form) on and in the body, but it simply does not get out of control due to the body's normally functioning immune system.

There are a number of reasons why candidiasis has become so much more common over the past thirty to forty years. The most important reason is probably the introduction of broad spectrum antibiotics at the end of the war. Other factors are the widespread use of the contraceptive pill, the use of steroids in various chronic illnesses and changes in our diet, mostly involving the consumption of large amounts of sugar and sugar containing foods. Certainly the pollution of our food chain with chemical pesticides and insecticides as well as the almost ubiquitous air pollution in the industrialized world must be other factors.

Unlike other infections and infestations it is difficult to prove whether candidiasis is present or not using conventional tests. This is because candida is present in the body to some extent in all of us. Because it is so widely found in nature, doctors and microbiologists alike take little notice of it. So therefore this is one of the very few instances where treatment is the main means of confirming the diagnosis. In other words, if a specific anti-candida treatment is given and it works, it can be assumed by inference that the original problem was due to a candidiasis. But could this simply be a placebo effect? We prefer testing for candida using the Vegatest system, but already through the history and clinical examination we have built up a strong index of suspicion that candida may be the primary problem.

Recently we have been considering a blood test known as the glucose fermentation test which looks at the capacity of candida, which is a yeast-like organism, to ferment sugar and produce alcohol. This can be detected in the blood. A blood test is taken to measure blood alcohol. The patient is then given 5 grammes of glucose (sugar) to ingest. An hour later another blood test is taken. If alcohol is present in the blood in the second test and none was found in the first test, this indicates that fermentation has gone on which is presumed to have been due to candida. We have found this test to be reliable, and it has produced no false positives, but unfortunately it does produce false negatives, that is patients who on the basis of successful treatment using an anti-candida approach have a negative glucose fermentation test.

So it is not foolproof, but it is the first test which is likely to be accepted by conventional medicine. The majority of conventional doctors consider the idea of candidal infestation apart from local infestation such as in the vagina, as being largely a figment of the imagination of doctors and therapists working within complementary medicine. This is because no test can be found to which conventional doctors can relate that proves it as present. Hopefully the glucose fermentation test is the first of a number of tests which will convince our conventional colleagues that candidal infestation is an important and growing problem.

It is important to remember that any yeast-like organism, given the right conditions, is capable of almost explosive growth, as anyone who has made bread will testify. The intestine is an ideal environment for this to happen because it is hot and moist. Normally candida is oval in shape, but there is accumulating evidence that in the body it adopts a mycelial form. We have been in contact with scientists working with fungi (mycologists) and they inform us that candida can survive quite happily in the intestine in the mycelial form.

In the mycelial form candida assumes a very complex branching structure, the individual branches being very fine and in some cases very long indeed, and these branches are called hyphae. They are extremely adept at passing between cell boundaries and opening up intercellular boundaries. If they do this in the gut lining, the net effect is that the gut lining behaves like a sieve in which the holes are too big, and toxins from the intestine are reabsorbed back into the liver through the local circulation (known as the portal circulation). The liver is often under stress anyway, particularly if the patient has a post viral syndrome. This then even further depletes the liver enzymes, and is the reason why treatment of the liver is a very important adjunct in the treatment of candida. In our experience complex homoeopathic preparations are the best means of doing this, together with avoidance of red meat, alcohol, coffee and fatty foods.

Our impression clinically is that in a very few patients candida in the mycelial form spreads throughout the lymphatic system as well. One particular patient when she got better, seemed to gradually clear up ascending up the legs and the abdomen and ended up with the last symptoms in the head. Our only possible conclusion was that the mycelial form of candida had spread throughout her lymphatic system.

The main indicators as to the presence of candidiasis are the symptoms. If you have five or more of these symptoms you are very likely to have candidiasis.

Abdominal bloating.

Intestinal gas, due to fermentation of sugars by the yeast-like candida organisms in the gut.

Loose stools.

A white itchy discharge which is in fact the candida coming out of the intestine, in the same way as when vaginal candida is present giving a white itchy discharge.

Itching, practically anywhere on the body.

Nail changes of both finger and toe nails giving thickened pitted nails, which often become grossly deformed, especially on the big toe.

Other fungal infestations such as athletes' foot, indicating the possibility that candidiasis is also present.

Excessive tiredness often unrelieved by rest.

Other less important indicators of candidiasis, but nevertheless common symptoms, are: irritability; inability to concentrate; depression and mood swings; numbness, tingling and weakness; weak muscles; heartburn; abdominal pain; recurrent sore throats; nasal congestion; swelling and discomfort in the joints; blurred vision; symptoms worsening in damp weather. The latter underlines the common association of candidiasis with sensitivity to airborne fungi (see Chapter 8).

Candida gets out of hand for a number of reasons, some already mentioned. They are as follows:

Underlying or inherited deficiency of the immune system such as post viral syndrome or Aids.

Aftermath of steroids taken in food (mostly meat), or as a medication.

As a result of taking the contraceptive pill in some women.

After taking antibiotics as a medication or in food, particularly in meat.

In diabetes.

In some cases of stress, particularly in any situation where there is constant or repeated states of anxiety, which results in depletion of vital reserves of nutrient that leads to immune depression. It can be shown that during stress the immune system works at a lower efficiency and there is increased usage of vital nutrients such as zinc and vitamin C (see Chapter 17).

CASE HISTORY

Susan is 36 years old, married with two children and works part-time. At 25 she began to notice increasing tiredness, lassitude, recurrent abdominal bloating, some abdominal pain, a white itchy discharge from the anus, and occasional loose bowels. Sometimes the tiredness was so severe that she simply had to lie down for an hour. In the past she has had three episodes of several vaginal thrush, which occurred whilst she was on the contraceptive pill. She is now no longer on the pill, but is aware that her libido has completely disappeared, causing problems in her marriage. She also has chronic catarrh which is significantly worse when the weather is damp.

This lady has chronic intestinal candidiasis, probably initially precipitated by the contraceptive pill. She has gradually become worse and worse, and now has acquired sensitivity to airborne spores, as evidenced by her chronic catarrh. The treatment was to give her an anti-candida diet, which produced pleasing results. She was then given nystatin powder, and eventually bowel bacteria replacements when the candidiasis had disappeared as a result of the treatment with nystatin powder. When first given the nystatin powder she felt temporarily worse due to a candida die-back reaction. This reaction is due to the initial toxins produced by the extensive destruction of the candida organism, and normally persists for approximately five days after the introduction of medication. Gradually all her symptoms disappeared, and her libido was regained. She is now completely normal and healthy, but has to be very careful not to eat large amounts of food containing sugar and yeast. If she eats any food containing sugar and yeast when she is slightly below par, i.e. if she is tired or she has a cold (that means when the immune system is working at less than peak efficiency), then her symptoms recur in a mild form. She therefore only risks breaking her diet when she is feeling completely well.

How to treat candidiasis

Dietary approaches
The main principle in an anti-candida diet is to avoid all sugar and yeast containing foods (see Chapter 20). In avoiding sugar it is important to remember that there is hidden sugar in many foods. If the candidiasis is very bad you would have to avoid all dried and fresh fruit. Fresh fruit is very high in fructose (fruit sugar), particularly melons, satsumas, mangoes and pink fleshed grapefruit. This approach on its own can sort out a lot of candida problems.

It may be important to adhere to this diet for some months in order to get a good result. An occasional break won't be the end of the world, but if on breaking the diet even slightly symptoms such as bloating and itching return, this indicates that you ought to stick to your diet very strictly. Generally speaking the longer you keep to the diet the less problems are incurred when breaking it from time to time. In certain circumstances it is unwise to break the diet at all and this is when the immune system is likely to be depressed. This might be because of stress, or due to having a cold or anything which makes you feel generally below par.

Homoeopathic approaches to candida
We have had a considerable degree of success by giving patients homoeopathic potencies of candida. We have a range of potencies available for testing in order to see which potency that particular patient requires at that particular time. We often add a potency of borax as well, which seems to help. In addition we have found it very useful to support the liver for reasons mentioned above using complex homoeopathic preparations. Ordinary herbal preparations which are directed at the liver can also be very useful.

Bowel bacterial replacements
These will be discussed more fully in the next chapter. Replacing the normal bowel flora can help very much in eliminating candida. The more friendly bacteria there are in the bowel the better.

Drug treatment for candida
In many cases the candidiasis is so severe that the only thing that will work is wholesale destruction of candida in the body using antifungal drugs. There are a number of these available of which the cheapest and probably the best is nystatin. This is derived from streptomyces, which is a cross between a fungus and a bacteria. The best form to give nystatin in is the powder form, and not the liquid or the tablet form in which it is usually dispensed. The liquid and tablet forms both have sugar added, which often makes the nystatin worse than useless. The normal dose of nystatin powder is half a teaspoon twice a day, but the dose can be increased depending on the severity of the candidiasis. One of the problems with nystatin powder is that it has a most unpleasant taste and some patients feel nauseous on taking it, but a high proportion of patients are able to take it. It is only available on prescription from doctors.

Fungilin is a commonly used antifungal, which is available in tablet form. It is highly effective and usually given as a dose of 100 mg four times a day. Certain other antifungals are important from time to time in cases in which nystatin and/or fungilin have failed. The most recent addition is a drug called diflucan, given 50 mg daily for seven days. It is important to take care with diflucan and other more potent antifungals such as nizoral, as they can cause liver damage. Therefore they can only be obtained on a doctor's prescription.

One important feature of the administration of these antifungals is that they must be given for a long period of time. In conventional medicine antifungals are usually only given for one week. This is worse than useless. Antifungals ought to be continued for at least two months in the first instance and probably longer. A number of conventional doctors refuse to look at the clinical evidence for this, but there is no doubt whatsoever in our minds that long courses of antifungals are absolutely essential.

All of the antifungals mentioned diminish the effectiveness of any bowel bacteria replacement (see Chapter 15), which is taken at the same time. There is however a more gentle antifungal known as caprilic acid which can be given at the same time as a bowel bacteria replacement. It ought however to be administered at a different time of the day. Our normal practice is to give caprilic acid 680 mg twice daily before meals with the bowel bacteria replacement taken between meals or first thing in the morning and last thing at night. Some patients also feel nauseous on taking caprilic acid.

Many people feel temporarily worse on taking antifungals, due to a so-called 'die-back' reaction, caused by the body having to deal with such large numbers of dead candida organisms that this can often overwhelm its ability to do so temporarily.

Other measures
If the patient is living in a damp house where his or her exposure to fungi is bound to be more than one would like, then if possible this situation ought to be rectified. Also desensitization to airborne fungal spores should be looked at.

Conclusion

Candidiasis is an increasingly common problem. It underlies many common chronic illnesses which we see in many cases of multiple food and chemical sensitivity. It needs to be treated very vigorously, and this involves a lot of co-operation from the patient as the dietary avoidance regime is not easy to follow.

CHAPTER 15

Dysbiosis – an unrecognized epidemic

Dysbiosis, sometimes called dysbacteria, is a condition in which abnormal intestinal bacteria are present. It is very common and it is largely unrecognized by conventional medicine. Normal bowel bacteria (known as bacterial flora) are 95% anaerobic – this means that they do not use oxygen and are killed on contact with oxygen. They mainly consist of the following types: bacteriodes, bacterium bifidum, various strains of escherichia coli, enterococci and lactobacilli. Proteus, yeasts, clostridia, staphylococci and aerobic spore producers are found in small numbers. These organisms form a symbiotic relationship, a biological relationship in which both host and bacteria benefit, with the colon, and the consequence of the absence of bacteria has been clearly demonstrated by experiments with animals reared in germ-free environments. Such animals soon succumb to fatal infection when released into the normal environment and show gross underdevelopment of their immune systems.

Symptom complex of dysbiosis

Symptoms are usually intestinal, such as flatulence, disordered bowel habit and intermittent abdominal swelling.

Theories on the subject of dysbiosis are legion and unfortunately often contradictory. Dysbiosis covers the symptom complexes of irritable bowel syndrome, spastic colon, ulcerative colitis and in some cases of Crohn's disease. Dysbiosis also underlies many cases of candidiasis, which in turn underlies much food sensitivity. The concept of dysbiosis seems to be a peculiarly German one, but for all that it is an eminently practical approach to an exceptionally common problem.

Relationships of the bacterial flora

There appears to be a physiological symbiotic balance between the acidophilus-bifidum group of bacteria and the coliform organisms (escherichia coli). If the coliform bacteria dominate then there is a tendency for the flora to rise in the intestine towards the small intestine. If the acidophilus-bifidum group (which are known as lactic acid fermenters) predominate, then the coliform bacteria are no longer able to function properly and the optimal colonic pH (a measure of acidity-alkalinity), which must be slightly alkaline, is changed because of the excess acid production of the lactic acid fermenter organisms. It should therefore be possible to treat dysbiosis with either preparations of coliform organisms or of acidophilus organisms.

The average healthy adult's intestine contains approximately 3 lbs of bacteria, this is equivalent to eleven to twelve trillion micro-organisms. Therefore to restore equilibrium when the body has been invaded by unfriendly bacteria requires literally billions and billions of viable, healthy lactobacillus acidophilus and bifido bacteria.

The ratio of lactobacillus acidophilus to bifido bacteria in the intestine depends on dietary habit. In most Westerners lactobacillus acidophilus predominate in the small intestine and bifido bacteria in the large. Vegans, or strict vegetarians, and certain ethnic groups tend to respond better to higher levels of bifido bacteria. This is explained by the fact that diets higher in complex carbohydrates support the growth of bifido bacteria.

Most importantly there appears to be a relationship between the permeability of the internal gut lining and normal bowel flora. If the flora is abnormal or unbalanced, then the gastro-intestinal mucous membrane becomes abnormally permeable, rather like a sieve in which the holes are too big, so allowing the absorption of inadequately broken down proteins and the re-absorption of toxins from the bowel contents.

Candida, as mentioned in the previous chapter, simply compounds this situation. This is often what happens in food sensitivity, and in our experience dysbiosis is a major underlying cause of such sensitivity. Simply treating the dysbiosis can result in the eventual disappearance of the majority of food sensitivities in patients who react to a variety of foods.

The toxins and proteins absorbed from the gut enter the liver circulation (the portal circulation) and may produce pharmacological effects due to the proteins being absorbed directly from the bowel into the blood stream. Normally proteins are not absorbed as whole molecules but rather as their individual amino-acids. Toxic effects also occur due to re-absorbed toxins from the gut.

This goes some way towards explaining why the simultaneous administration of a liver remedy is useful when treating dysbiosis.

Causes of dysbiosis

The most common cause is antibiotic usage. This may be antibiotics given medicinally or taken in food, particularly meat. As a result the colonic flora is damaged in many people. A proportion of patients regain their normal bacteria, especially if they are sensible enough to take plenty of live yoghurt following a course of antibiotics. However, it is unclear why yoghurt should help restore the normal bacterial flora, if indeed it does, as it contains lactobacillus bulgaricus and not lactobacillus acidophilus. Lactobacillus acidophilus does not even survive well in yoghurt. The best alternative is to take a course of lactobacillus acidophilus obtained from a health food shop.

Other factors which cause dysbiosis are poor nutrition, particularly the consumption of large quantities of junk food, and severe illness which causes a large outpouring of toxins discharged from the body via the colon, which can upset the flora. Clearly any enteritis (infective diarrhoea), will by its very nature upset the normal bacterial population.

Functional and organic disease of the gastro-intestinal tract together with dysfunction of the liver and pancreas commonly go hand in hand with dysbiosis, which should therefore be looked for in cases of hepatitis or pancreatitis. Pancreatic or liver dysfunction will upset the gastro-intestinal pH (the acid/alkaline level), which is critical for the gut flora to function normally. Without it, the stomach creates too much acid (as in hyper-acidic gastritis) and then the alkaline bile, pancreatic and small intestinal excretions are not sufficient to neutralize the excess gastric acid. As a result digestion is incomplete and becomes subject to fermentation processes, particularly if there is excess carbohydrate intake. In these situations there will be a lot of gas production and abdominal distension. If protein forms a large part of the diet then there will be putrification with foul smelling intestinal gas. In both cases an excess of bacterial colonization of the bowel will occur and consequently this increases fermentation or putrification, depending on whether the diet predominates in carbohydrates or proteins, which in the end will produce a dysbacteria.

Stress, a ubiquitous cause of many illnesses, affects the gastro-intestinal lining membrane, which can in turn cause changes in the normal gut flora leading to an invasion of bacteria foreign to the intestine.

Normal function of the bowel flora

Bowel bacteria are essential to the development of the normal immune system, as experiments with germ-free animals have shown. In these animals the weight and length of the small intestine, for example, is reduced, as is the lymphatic system.

Intestinal bacteria can synthesize vitamins, mostly the B group but also vitamin K. In dysbiosis the majority of vitamins taken by mouth, either in food or by vitamin replacement, will be taken up by the abnormal bacteria, resulting in vitamin deficiency. This may well be why large doses of vitamins are found to be effective, whereas low doses are often useless. Orthomolecular medicine, which has as its hallmark the administration of megadoses of vitamins and minerals, has been based on this observation. Our suggestion is that if the underlying dysbiosis was adequately treated then smaller doses of vitamins would be adequate.

The diagnosis of dysbiosis

The history is the most important pointer, but it will not be obvious if dysbiosis is present as a hidden underlying cause of chronic illness. Post viral syndrome, acne, candidiasis, asthma, urticaria, eczema and rheumatism are the most common diseases which have dysbiosis as a possible underlying cause. Constipation, flatulence, morning diarrhoea or any irregular bowel habit, foul smelling faeces, intermittent abdominal swelling, all point to a possible dysbiosis. The diagnosis could also be made by bacteriological examination of the faeces. In practice this is laborious and expensive due to the fact that most bowel organisms are anaerobic, and so have to be grown in special cabinets from which the air has been excluded.

CASE HISTORY

John is a 53 year old ex-college lecturer who had to take early retirement due to his illness. He has been a smoker all his life, but has given up recently. Ten years ago he developed recurrent chronic bronchitis which needed many courses of antibiotics. He gradually found that he became more and more under par, between his courses of antibiotics, yet his chest remained clear at these times. His abdomen started to bloat, and his bowel habit became irregular. Stopping smoking had little effect on these symptoms. He developed abdominal wind, sometimes had abdominal pain and his symptoms became so bad that he had to apply for early retirement.

We treated him by first of all getting rid of the candidiasis present in his bowel using an anti-candida diet and nystatin powder. We then replaced his normal bowel bacteria, with a mixture of bacteria mostly containing human strain lactobacillus acidophilus, as he is not a vegetarian. It took several months of this bowel bacteria replacement and simultaneous treatment of his liver with a complex homoeopathic preparation, but he gradually regained his earlier health, and is now perfectly well and healthy. Having stopped smoking he no longer gets recurrent chronic bronchitis and therefore no longer needs to resort to regular courses of antibiotics. When he does get a chest infection he immediately treats himself with large doses of vitamin C, that is 4 grammes three times daily, together with a classical homoeopathic remedy, which so far has kept him away from using antibiotics.

The treatment of dysbiosis

The mainstays of treatment are replacing the normal flora by using preparations of bacteria in suspended animation. They are supplied in packs in a dormant state. On exposure to heat or moisture, the bacteria re-animate and quickly lose their potency if not put straight into a suitable environment such as the intestinal tract. The better the bowel bacteria replacement the higher the bacterial count, measured in terms of millions of organisms per gramme.

The actual bacteria in the bowel bacteria replacement is of fundamental importance. The majority of preparations are lactobacillus acidophilus or bifido bacteria. Some patients need a higher percentage of bifido bacteria, and others need a higher percentage of lactobacillus acidophilus. Generally speaking vegans, Asians and others on a high complex carbohydrate diet need 80% bifido bacteria and 20% lactobacillus acidophilus. Individuals on a normal Western diet would require 80% lactobacillus acidophilus and 20% bifido bacteria.

Recently there has been a great deal of work on what the ideal strains of bacteria would be to repopulate the bowel. Veterinary work has clearly shown that giving species-specific bacteria yields very much better results than non-species-specific bacteria. What is found is that the species-specific bacteria sticks much more readily to the gut lining. Practically all human bowel bacteria replacement sold at the present time is not human species-specific. This probably means that a large number of them do not stick to the gut lining and are excreted in the faeces. Coupled with the fact that, as they are taken by mouth, gastric acid would kill off 70% of them anyway, this means there is a case in severe cases of dysbacteria for implanting the bowel bacteria directly into the colon. This is often done after giving a colonic wash-out, which is a form of treatment which often helps in cases of dysbiosis and in candidiasis. In our view simply giving the patient a vigorous purge over two or three days during which time they have diarrhoea, produces as good a clinical result as a colonic wash-out, and is a lot cheaper.

Recently one manufacturer of bowel bacteria replacement has introduced some human species-specific bacteria and, in our opinion, this preparation is more clinically effective. Undoubtedly this is because a species-specific strain of bacteria is much more likely to stick to the gut lining and then to divide in the gut and re-establish a normal bacterial population. There are tens of thousands of strains of the various bacteria referred to in this chapter present in the bowel. It is therefore important to get the strains right, but at the moment this is not a practical possibility. One possible development of this is that it may be possible in the future to culture specific strains from patients' stools and establish exactly what strains that particular patient requires, so that each patient would get a specific collection of suitable strains. We would anticipate that this would lead to much more effective treatment of a whole host of chronic illnesses.

CHAPTER 16

Post viral syndrome or myalgic encephalomyelitis (ME)

Post viral syndrome and myalgic encephalomyelitis (ME) are important underlying causes of multiple food sensitivity. They are currently the subject of much debate in medical literature and the lay media. The question being asked by both the medical profession and the public is 'Is this a genuine illness?'.

The typical history is a viral infection usually with 'flu-like symptoms, glandular fever or occasionally stomach upset with diarrhoea and vomiting. Following the viral infection there is not a complete return to health. This is usually accompanied by a large number of symptoms, the most common being persistent tiredness, lethargy and lack of energy characteristically unrelieved by sleep. The sleep pattern itself tends to change, and often is abnormally deep and long, yet unrefreshing. In some other cases it becomes broken and disturbed. Muscle pain is often very severe, most commonly in the legs, and often made worse by exercise. This is a common feature of ME in particular, but not so common in other post viral syndromes. It is important to point out here that ME is one of a number of post viral syndromes, which may be due to viruses such as Epstein-Barr, coxsackie or related viruses, or may be due to emotional and psychological stress in conjunction with a viral infection.

The resulting physical debility is often matched by psychological symptoms such as loss of short term memory, inability to concentrate and uncharacteristic emotional lability. Often the regulation of sweating, heart rate, body temperature and digestive processes of various kinds seem to be out of sync. This would imply that the virus attacks the centre of the autonomic nervous system in the brain, the nervous system which governs our internal body functions, called the hypothalamus.

Even minimal stress, both physical and psychological, characteristically worsens the symptoms and not surprisingly depression is common. The worst sufferers are confined to bed for weeks at a time.

This bewildering array of symptoms often elicits an unsympathetic response from doctors. Coupled with this there is often manifest multiple food and chemical sensitivity which compounds the problem as far as the patient is concerned, as they are very much given the feeling that they are not genuinely ill. The last straw is that there is no conventional medical blood test, rather like in candidiasis, which can confirm whether the patient has post viral syndrome or ME or is malingering. One recent test has been developed which is called a viral protein 1 test, and looks for antibodies to certain viruses in the body, particularly enteroviruses. These are viruses which attack the intestine. It is interesting to note that polio is an enterovirus. This test has been found to be positive in approximately 24% of patients suffering from ME, but if the test turns out negative, it does not necessarily mean that the patient is malingering.

Because so little is understood about these illnesses there is a range of terms used to describe them such as myalgic encephalomyelitis (ME), post viral syndrome (PVS), post viral fatigue syndrome (PVFS), chronic fatigue syndrome (CFS) and chronic fatigue and immunodeficiency syndrome (CFIDS). All these terms refer to the same disorder.

Post viral syndromes are now the subject of much research. There have been recent interesting findings, which are more helpful in terms of establishing the causes of this increasingly widespread problem – informed sources have claimed that there are probably more than a quarter of a million sufferers in the United Kingdom alone. One of the more interesting has been the demonstration of viral particles inside cells destroying the mitochondria which are the 'engines' of the cell. It is no wonder that patients with post viral syndrome have so little energy!

The range of viruses thought to be involved in post viral syndrome are the entero viruses, coxsackie virus, the 'flu viruses, and the Epstein-Barr virus which is a herpes virus causing glandular fever. Unfortunately looking for raised blood levels of antibodies to these viruses is not particularly helpful. For example a recent study looked at levels of antibodies to the coxsackie virus in patients with clinical post viral syndrome and compared them with the normal population. There was no difference. Also as far as the Epstein-Barr virus is concerned the vast majority of the population has been infected with this virus subclinically (in other words, had the illness but has not had any symptoms, like for example German measles which is a similar illness and often produces only a slight rash and no other symptoms) and therefore 90% of us have antibodies to it. A good deal of current work on post viral syndromes has been devoted to looking at the immune systems of those patients who get this illness syndrome, to see whether there is anything different about their immune systems which means that they react to these viruses in a different way to the majority of the population.

ME and post viral syndrome are therefore illnesses of the immune system as a whole and do not fit in with the current medical philosophy of illness, which seeks to put diseases into separate compartments and demands that each disease should fit into only one single compartment. It also tries to identify a single cause for each disease and to direct treatment at the elimination of this single cause. This leads the conventional medical approach to devote much of its attention to alleviating symptoms without addressing the patient's general situation at a more holistic level.

This is why the discovery that the immune system is very much affected by emotional factors, which has given birth to the science of psychoneuro-immunology, has been a major step forward, because it means that conditions like ME can be approached concurrently on an emotional and on a physical level (see Chapter 17). Therefore in a real sense ME and post viral syndromes can be considered as a disorder of the mind and body, but without implying that the patient is somehow emotionally weak and has caused his own problem. This is a stigma which is going to be very slow to disappear, as many patients will still feel that if the emotions are addressed from a treatment point of view, the disease is somehow their fault.

Looking at stress is often a primarily important factor in confirming vulnerability to infection with viruses which are relatively harmless to most of us, such as the glandular fever virus. It may be this that is making the patient who does develop post viral syndrome react differently to the virus from other people who do not. It is therefore significant that many patients with post viral syndrome are found to have suffered a period of stress at or around the time of the initial viral infection. This might have been a bereavement, a divorce, a loss of job, etc.

The treatment of post viral syndrome

Identification of food sensitivity is an important first step, as it relieves much of the stress on the immune system. Then attending to the almost universal intestinal candidiasis and dysbiosis also produces pleasing results. Looking at the patient's mineral and vitamin state is as important, as often the enzyme systems of these patients are very much depleted, and rectifying marked deficiencies of zinc and magnesium amongst others (see Chapter 11) produces useful results. A recent double blind study carried out by one of us showed that magnesium supplementation by intramuscular injection of magnesium sulphate was significantly effective in improving patients with ME. Lastly complex homoeopathic therapy directed mainly at supporting the liver and detoxifying the body, together with stress reducing approaches such as psychotherapy, a body work technique or whatever happens to suit that particular patient, completes the treatment picture.

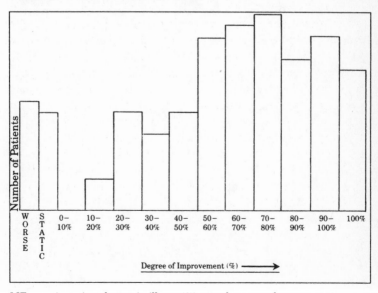

ME questionnaire: change in illness (%) over three months treatment.

In our own Centre where we use this broad-based approach, we find that approximately 50% of our patients get 70% better (assessed on a questionnaire) over a course of treatment. We followed up the patients over a three month period to come to these conclusions. The graph on page 169 and list of results below summarizes our findings.

Our conclusion is that post viral syndrome and ME are not untreatable illnesses, and looking at them in a holistic way can produce very significant and long-lasting clinical improvements.

ME Questionnaire – Results

1.	Sex ratio:	Sent: Male 24% Female 76%
		Replies: Male 24% Female 86%
2.	Age range:	7 to 64 years Average 37.5%
		(90% between 15 and 55 years)
3.	Racial origins:	*No* Non-Caucasians
4.	Locality of home:	No significant factors
5.	Positive V.P.1:	24%
6.	Duration of illness:	6 months to 12 years

CHAPTER 17

Emotional causes of multiple sensitivity

Conventional medicine has very much divided mind and body into two separate compartments. Somehow mind or emotionally caused illnesses are not real. This is beginning to change, as researchers in the field of immunology have been observing for some years the influence of various psychological processes on immune responses. These observations indicate that there must be communication between the nervous system and the immune system. Gradually out of this the science of psychoneuro-immunology was born. Recently interest in this new area of medicine has burgeoned, and at the Seventh International Congress of Immunology in Berlin in August 1989 there were more than 160 papers dealing with interactions between the immune and nervous systems.

The immune system is a highly interconnected system, communicating by a whole variety of molecules, some like antibodies and some like hormones, and it contains many feedback paths to regulate itself. Superimposed upon this is a complex set of communications between the immune system and the nervous system. Most of the immunological hormone-like molecules (called lymphokines), which are a very important means of communication between white cells, have many effects within the body, many of them in the nervous system. Conversely, all of the active nervous system chemicals in the body which act as mediators from one nerve cell to another have been found to influence the immune response in some way. It is not possible to separate mind from body, therefore the immune system reacts to any emotion whatever it is.

Stress

Highly significant connections have been found between stress, immune depression and susceptibility to viral infections, auto-immune diseases or cancer. The types of stress studied have included bereavement, unemployment, marital trauma and university examinations. What has been found is that it is not the stress itself which affects the immune response, but the way the person perceives that stress. In other words, what is stressful to one person may not worry another. This is why 'good copers' are less prone to the immune effects of stress. It also shows clearly that our thoughts and feelings do influence our susceptibility to a wide range of disease, and how altering the way we respond to stress can fundamentally affect the way we respond to illness.

Conditioning of immune responses

It has been found that it is possible to train the immune system to respond in a conditioned way, in the same way that Pavlov trained his dogs to respond by salivating simply by ringing a bell. He first associated food with bell ringing, until ultimately the food was withdrawn and the bell was merely rung to initiate salivation in the dog. Recently work has been done with rats administering an immunosuppressive drug at the same time as sweetened drinking water. Soon sweetened drinking water on its own was enough to damp the immune response in these animals.

It is very likely that the placebo effect is a conditioned immune response in which subjects given a remedy containing no medicinally active compound believe and respond as if they are taking an active medicament. It is also known that strongly held beliefs and expectations can dramatically alter immune processes. All these facts open up all sorts of possibilities for treating immune suppression leading to multiple sensitivities, by doing such things as altering the way people react to stress, especially looking at how they perceive stress.

A number of conventional doctors have suggested that multiple food and chemical sensitivities are due to emotionally caused hyperventilation, and that the patients can simply be treated by telling them to breathe into a paper bag held over the face, which has the effect of increasing blood levels of carbon dioxide, in order to correct their hyperventilation. It is possible to monitor as to whether the patient is over-breathing on sophisticated conventional respiratory measurement apparatus. It is in fact true that a number of multiply sensitive patients do hyperventilate. The way to treat them is to address the underlying emotional cause, as well as teach them slower deeper abdominal breathing. This does work well for a small proportion of emotionally caused multiple sensitivities. It does not mean, as some conventional doctors have suggested, that *all* multiply sensitive patients are neurotic hyperventilators.

Treatment

Homoeopathy has a lot to offer for emotional problems. The mainstays are Bach flower remedies or high potency single homoeopathics. Bach flower remedies can be self-administered, and appropriate repertories together with medications (there are thirty-eight Bach flower remedies, all derived from a variety of indigenous flowers) are available from most health food shops. High potency classical single homoeopathic remedies only ought to be given by a competent, experienced and qualified practitioner.

In many cases the homoeopathic approach will bring to the surface the relevant feelings, and these can be acted out, and understood, with appropriate resolution of the emotional problem. Our own practice is to often accompany this with psychotherapy or a body work technique (our choice is biodynamic massage) as a means of helping the patient reach and experience and understand the feelings underlying the problem. Psychotherapy, which is a talking approach, suits some patients, others need a more physical body work technique in order to really get into the feelings and discharge them.

So often the multiple sensitivities which the patient displays are surface manifestations of often deeply buried emotional conflicts. The important thing is that the patient is given a therapy which helps them dig down beneath the surface and reach and understand these problems. Only then can they be properly discharged and resolved.

CASE HISTORY

Mrs M. came to see us complaining of extreme sensitivity to tapwater, to the extent that she was unable to drink any, and could hardly put any on her skin. This adverse reaction to water followed a severe gastroenteritis which she contracted in September 1980. She had also developed a wide range of food sensitivities.

Her underlying problem was one of dysbiosis with a secondary candidiasis, together with a large number of toxins accumulating in the liver. We treated her from that point of view using preparations directed at the liver, bowel bacteria replacement, and desensitizing her to tap water. She was so sensitive to water that the diluent (i.e. the substance in which the drops were diluted), had to be highly purified water, and we had to use de-ionised water from a cancer research laboratory. If the wrong diluent was put in by accident, she would be able to recognize it consistently, on a blind basis, in other words she would have no idea as to whether we had made a mistake or not. Once or twice we purposely made a mistake to see whether she could pick it out and indeed every time she did so. Her condition reached a fairly tolerable level, but she continued to need drops.

On enquiring into her previous history, it turned out that as a young child of five she was dangled over a bridge over a fast running deep river by an older child. She was naturally terrified. When she was nine her father committed suicide by jumping off a bridge into running water. Then at the age of ten she fell into a deep stream trying to retrieve a toy for a friend of hers, and she was unable to swim. Not surprisingly she became pathologically frightened of water.

We decided to treat her along this line, and a hypnotherapist would regress her on a number of occasions back to these traumatic events. On reliving and acting out the fear, terror and panic which these incidents brought about, she has gradually been able to dispense with all the homoeopathic medications and the desensitization drops, and is slowly returning to normal.

This is a very clear example of a conditioned immune response, entirely emotionally caused. It is very easy to miss that, particularly since as a therapist it is easy to get bogged down in the technology of food and chemical sensitivity, in other words desensitization drops, homoeopathic treatment, etc., etc. It needs a wise physician to be able to dig beneath the surface to find the basic underlying cause of any patient's problem, and this particular case is very illustrative of this situation.

In the final analysis the patient, if he or she is willing to, can ask questions as to what their illness is telling them, what it means to them in their life journey, and how best to see it as a learning experience. This sort of attitude is by far the most constructive approach to emotionally-based multiple food and chemical sensitivities. So often patients end up with a feeling of guilt that somehow it is all their fault, which more often than not does not lead to any constructive approach, merely to antidepressants and tranquillizers, often being prescribed for many years.

CHAPTER 18

Multiply sensitive patients

It is increasingly common for a very small number of people to react to a very wide range of foods and chemicals. They have been called universal reactors. These people are very difficult indeed to treat, and life is practically impossible for them, let alone their close relatives. There are two ways of handling this situation.

The first is to be admitted to an ecology unit. This is a unit in which all the building materials are environmentally safe, all the food is organic, and a wide variety of diets is catered for. Everybody coming in to the building is screened and certainly nobody is allowed to wear any perfume or strongly smelling make-up. In this sort of protected environment many universal reactors improve markedly.

There are a number of practical disadvantages to this approach. The first one is that ecology units are extremely expensive to run. This means that the cost to the patient will be in the order of £300 or more per day. Clearly this would only be available to patients who have full private health insurance, or who are very well off. From a medical point of view, once patients leave this sort of unit they are out into the outside world again, and find it even more difficult to adapt than they did before they went in. So some patients find themselves even more sensitive. It could therefore be argued on medical grounds alone, that ecology units can cause more problems than they solve. They are relatively popular in America, and in this country there are two ecology units.

When patients are in an ecology unit it is possible to carry out a range of treatments which would be difficult to give on a regular basis when the patient is seen as an out-patient. These techniques are used on an out-patient basis in some clinics, but often cannot be given often enough in order to have sufficiently marked clinical effect. The treatments consist of intravenous administration of minerals and vitamins. The vitamin given intravenously is most commonly vitamin C, and sometimes B group vitamins are added. Intravenous minerals used are most commonly magnesium and zinc, and less commonly chromium and selenium. Some clinics make extensive use of hydrogen peroxide drips, for which they claim great success in the treatment of candidiasis. Also colonic wash-outs are sometimes used as a means of detoxifying the patient.

The other more practical approach to universal reactors is to search for underlying causes and treat these underlying causes vigorously. The most common underlying causes are post viral syndromes of various sorts, and emotional problems. It is only the most experienced practitioners, with a wide range of therapies available to them, who can cope with these sort of cases with any degree of success. Often they take a number of years to recover and in the end may still have to cope with a fairly limited lifestyle. As universal reactors are becoming more common, it is important that practical means of managing their problems are increasingly widely available.

CASE HISTORY

John is a 31 year old accountant who contracted a severe viral illness two years ago. The symptoms of the virus were generalized body aching, an intermittent temperature, and slight diarrhoea. The initial infection lasted approximately two weeks. He then began to feel slightly better but never regained his original levels of energy. He found that gradually more and more foods produced a wide range of symptoms including generalized aches, headaches, some foods causing diarrhoea and some causing a blocked-up nose. He soon was restricted to eating chicken, boiled swede and buckwheat only. His energy levels had reached an all-time low, to the extent that he was confined to bed twenty-four hours a day. Not being married he had to move back to his parents' home in order to be looked after.

John was admitted to an ecology unit. He was desensitized for fifty-eight different foods, and found he was soon able to eat moderate amounts of a wide range of foods to which he was previously sensitive, using desensitization drops. It took approximately three weeks to determine the end points of all these foods, using the Miller technique (see Chapter 6). Once the desensitization levels had been determined, he received daily intravenous drips of vitamin C, supplemented with magnesium and B group vitamins which previous blood tests had shown he was deficient in. After a further three weeks in the ecology unit, he regained approximately 60% of his previous energy levels.

He left the unit on high oral doses of vitamin C, magnesium and the B group vitamins together with desensitization drops. He was soon able to return to work and was able to lead a relatively normal life, even though his energy levels were not as high as before his viral infection. He was also restricted to relatively small amounts of the foods to which he was desensitized.

CASE HISTORY

Shirley is a 42 year old mother of three. The family had moved to an old country cottage three years previously. The survey of the cottage showed that there was extensive wood-worm, and some dry rot. They were given a generous allowance on the price of the cottage, and planned to attend to these problems after having moved into the house. On moving in they contacted a company who eradicated the woodworm and dry rot using chemical treatments including lindane. The house was also fumigated. Whilst this was done, the family moved out into their small caravan for four days and then came back into the house.

A week later Shirley began to notice that she was developing headaches and her nose was running constantly. Gradually the headaches became more and more severe and she also started to react to household cleaning materials. She then found that her symptoms were much worse when she went in her car shopping to the local town, especially when she stopped to fill the car with petrol. The next thing she noticed was that she was unable to go to any pubs or any gathering where anybody was smoking. Cigarette smoke gave her intolerable headaches. Gradually her life became more and more restricted as she reacted to more and more chemicals, and on top of that she soon began to react to a wide range of common foods.

After seeing many specialists and doctors and getting no help of any sort, she was sent to an ecology unit. Specialized blood tests were carried out to measure the levels of pesticides in her blood and she was found to have high levels of a wide range of pesticides, including lindane. She was desensitized to a wide range of chemicals using the Miller technique. She found that this worked admirably, but only for two to three days. It was soon established that the desensitization end point was moving every three days, and so the painful series of injections to determine end points had to be repeated. Gradually, however, the desensitization end points settled down, and she was given intravenous vitamin and mineral therapy and regained some degree of normality to her life. After two months in the ecology unit she was discharged.

On getting back home, after only two days, she started reacting to a wide range of chemicals in spite of her desensitization. Her condition deteriorated, and she remains reacting to a wide range of chemicals, with energy levels approximately 50% of what they were before she was poisoned. In her case the ecology unit had been of some benefit, but she was unable to live for ever in such a highly protected environment. On going back into the normal world again, she soon found she was even more maladapted than before she went.

Subsequently she obtained some degree of benefit using homoeopathic methods for detoxifying, together with homoeopathic dilutions specially prepared of all the pesticides used when the house was treated. However it was not possible to improve her to anything like the levels of health she had before moving into their new house and having it treated for woodworm and dry rot.

CHAPTER 19

The dangers of clinical ecology

There are two dangers in an ecological approach to illness, firstly misdiagnosis and secondly malnutrition.

As an ecological approach to illness produces many startling clinical results, often quite quickly in chronic diseases which are otherwise very difficult to treat, this can lead practitioners, doctors and non-medically qualified practitioners alike to apply ecological methods over-enthusiastically, and thereby missing serious underlying problems. It is always safer to go to see a doctor practising ecology rather than a non-medical practitioner. This does not decry the skills of non-medically qualified ecologists, but they simply do not have the same clinical experience and clinical judgement to pick up what is always a difficult to diagnose underlying disease.

The commonest situation is a patient who has a basic underlying emotional problem masquerading as multiple food and chemical sensitivities. These can be very difficult patients to handle, as multiple food and chemical sensitivities give them something to put their symptoms on to, which means they do not need to look at their emotional or spiritual health. To correctly judge this requires a very balanced approach from the practitioner. Often it will need several consultations over a period of many months to properly assess what the patient's problem really is, and to decide what the most fruitful way forward is, based on how he or she responds to various treatments. In this type of case that might be using psychotherapy alone, with ecological treatments such as desensitization and diets merely acting as a back-up to smooth the patient's day to day existence as far as possible.

Malnutrition is the second danger in ecological treatment. The most serious risk is calcium deficiency due to elimination from the diet of high calcium containing foods, milk and dairy products, to which patients are very commonly sensitive. It is important to give a calcium supplement in these cases, particularly in children, and to encourage the consumption of other calcium-rich foods such as sardines, nuts, green vegetables, etc. Deficiency of B group vitamins can occur through the avoidance of yeast, and in rare cases iodine deficiency can be occasioned by the avoidance of milk, dairy products and fish. Make sure that whichever practitioner you go to has a good grasp of nutritional medicine, which would alert him to possible nutritional deficiencies as a result of dietary therapy.

A less serious consequence of ecological treatment is that it can create an environmental neurosis, which makes life a nightmare for the patient and his or her close relatives. If the patient is already introspective, then too much reliance on diets can worsen this problem, and make life absolutely impossible. In this situation it is best to concentrate on underlying causes. The practice of multiple desensitization using the Miller technique can also add to this environmental neurosis. It needs a well balanced practitioner to be able to judge this properly, so as to stop this situation developing. For example a practitioner will think twice before putting a young girl on a severely restricted diet if she has previously had a history of anorexia. A much more balanced approach would be to look at other ways of treating her migraine, for which there are many ways within complementary medicine, which do not run the risk of rekindling her anorexia.

Provided a balanced, non-partisan approach is adopted, none of these dangers need arise. However it bears pointing out that the dangers of ecological treatment pale into insignificance when compared with the dangers of conventional drug and surgical treatment. Practitioners of complementary medicine are being taken to task for complications which do occur, such as the dangers mentioned in this chapter, and the implication is that these dangers are widespread, whereas in fact they are not. However, within conventional medicine the iatrogenic (doctor caused) side effects are commonplace. Recent research suggests that the expected complication rate after operation, primarily due to medical incompetence, is 4% of patients admitted. This is a classic situation of looking for a speck in the eye of the complementary practitioner whilst ignoring the moat in one's own.

CHAPTER 20

Food exclusion diets

Introduction

The aim of this chapter is not to provide an exhaustive list of food alternatives. There are many diet books available that will help with specific recipes such as for sugar free, milk free, yeast free and wheat free cooking. Our aim is to give some general guiding principles as to how we feel a food exclusion diet is best managed, so that it will cause the minimum amount of inconvenience and difficulty, as well as being nutritionally adequate and ecologically safe.

It is our firm belief that individuals should not place themselves on food exclusion diets for prolonged periods of time without seeking nutritional advice through a competent practitioner or doctor. A number of people we have seen have placed themselves on very complex and restrictive dietary regimes. In some instances these have been quite clearly part of an eating disorder such as anorexia or bulaemia, in other cases the dietary restrictions have been the only way that food sensitive individuals have found themselves able to control their complex food intolerances.

If you find your diet is becoming increasingly complex and difficult to manage, then there may well be an underlying cause for the food intolerances, either physiological or psychological. You will not be able to broaden your diet unless this pathology is dealt with adequately, be it an eating disorder, intestinal candidiasis or a focus of infection such as a chronic appendicitis.

One of the first, and probably the most important, principles of all medical practice is that the treatment should not itself be harmful. We therefore believe very strongly that any dietary regime should take this into account whether it is self-imposed or suggested by a competent doctor or complementary medical practitioner. It is our usual practice to suggest a food exclusion diet for a month and then review both the clinical effects of this procedure and the nutritional status of the individual. We also offer telephone advice as part of our consultation procedure, if needed for individual patients. In spite of this we find that some people continue with their food exclusion diet without seeking further nutritional advice, even though we have done everything within our power to avoid this situation occurring.

What foods can I eat?

All food exclusion diets by their very nature involve a restrictive element. It is however very important that you have a clear list of the foods that you can eat. In some instances this general rule may be waived for a short period of time, for instance in the use of a five day fasting technique to isolate the foods to which you may be reacting. However the five day spring water fast should only be carried out under strict supervision as outlined in Chapter 10.

The standard testing systems which we use involves a biological measurement such as the Vegatest. This allows the practitioner to tell the patient which foods they should avoid, but also which can be eaten freely. The information given about the foods it is possible to eat is almost more valuable to the affected individual as it allows them to develop a coherent and nutritionally adequate dietary regime. The foods we test at the first consultation are:

Milk (cow's)	Beet sugar	Fish
Milk (goat's)	Molasses	Shellfish
Milk (sheep's)	Preservatives	Smoked fish
Cheese	Monosodium gluto-	Peas
Egg white	mate (E621)	Beans
Corn	Tartrazine (E102)	Sprouts
Wheat	Colourants (E104,	(brassicas)
Rye	107, 110, 122, 123,	Cabbage
Oats	124, 128, 150)	(brassicas)
Barley	Rice	Cauliflower
Coffee	Egg yolk	(brassicas)
Tea	Lemons	Beef
Chocolate (milk)	Mushrooms	Chicken
Chocolate (plain)	Yeast: live	Pork (inc. ham
Cocoa	Yeast: dead (yeast	and bacon)
Cane sugar	extract, bread)	Potatoes

Specific diseases associated with allergy

Tomatoes	Nuts	Sultanas
Oranges	Peanuts	Currants
Alcohol	Onions	Raisins
Potassium	Carrots	Lamb
Sodium (salt)	Apples	Turkey
Soya	Bananas	

While this is not an exhaustive list, it covers the vast majority of common foods. There will rarely be more than eight or ten foods to avoid, usually no more than two of the major foods (that is foods that are commonly used within other foods, such as wheat or milk). It is always important to consider the positive aspects of dietary restriction and to look at the interesting combinations that can be developed from the foods that need not be avoided. One of the main advantages of testing systems like the Vegatest and applied kinesiology are that they allow a clear decision to be made about the foods that are and are not tolerated.

Food rotation

Until fairly recently it has been very difficult for most of the population to become food addicted. Many of our foods are harvested seasonally, consequently over a period of a year the foods may be available in excess for some weeks or months and then unavailable for a much longer period of time. It is only with improved methods of food storage and far swifter transport systems that we have been able to have the same high quality fruits and vegetables consistently supplied to us throughout the year.

It is therefore now easy for us to develop food fads, only eating particular types of food for sustained periods of time. People who develop such 'food addictions' may well go on to develop intolerance to the foods which they eat persistently. As a general rule therefore, no one should continue to eat the same food day in and day out. If you have already demonstrated the potential to develop food intolerance it is particularly important that you rotate your foods; for instance your breakfast should sometimes involve cereal, sometimes toast and sometimes fruit, but not the same thing each morning.

Ideally you should try to rotate and vary your food on a two or three day basis. If you are at the stage where you are becoming more food tolerant, having been allergic, then you should reintroduce the once forbidden foods once every five or even once every seven days initially. If you eat previously forbidden foods on a daily basis you are quite likely to redevelop food intolerance to that particular food through the process of active sensitization (Chapter 10). Regular food rotation is therefore important for all of us, particularly those who have the propensity to develop food intolerances.

Sometimes various food families cross-react. For instance tomato and potato are part of the same food family. Peppers, chilli, tobacco and egg plants are also in this family. As a consequence somebody who has a food sensitivity to potatoes and tomatoes will often go on to develop sensitivity to green pepper and egg plant if these are eaten in excess. It must be stressed that cross-reactions within food families tend to occur only in particularly food sensitive individuals. Normally it is perfectly adequate to simply rotate the food without considering food families. It is however a point to bear in mind if you are a particularly food sensitive person and wish to plan a detailed food rotation.

As well as basing food families on their botanical relationship, they can also be categorized according to the chemicals they share. This has been explained in Chapter 9. In our experience, in particularly sensitive individuals, there is a clear potential for foods to cross-react both within their food families and within their phenolic group. It is important to stress however that unless an individual is particularly food sensitive there is no over-riding necessity to take account of food families or phenolic groups in their initial management. We have, however, included the food families both for the sake of completeness and for those few individuals who may need them. It is not our intention to make food exclusions more complex than they need be!

Food families
Apple family: apple, cider, cider vinegar, pectin, pear, quince, quince seed.
Arrowroot family: arrowroot.
Arum family: taro, poi, dasheen.
Banana family: banana, plantain.
Birch family: filbert, hazel nut.
Brazil family: Brazil nut.
Buckwheat family: buckwheat, rhubarb, garden sorrel.
Cactus family: cactus, tequila, prickly pear.

Caper family: capers.

Carob family.

Cashew family: cashew, pistachio, mango.

Cereal family: corn meal, corn starch, corn oil, corn sugar (syrup, dextrose, glucose, cerelose), wheat flour, bran, wheat germ, farina, barley, malt, rye, oats, rice, wild rice, sorghum, cane sugar, molasses, bamboo shoots, millet.

Chicory family: chicory.

Citrus family: orange, grapefruit, lemon, lime, tangerine, kumquat, citron, citrange, angostura.

Cochliospernum family: gum karaya, gum guaiac.

Composite family: leaf lettuce, head lettuce, endive, escarole, artichoke, dandelion, chicory, oyster plant salsify, celtuse, sunflower seeds (seed oil, sesame seed oil), absinthe, vermouth (cragweed, pyrethrum).

Ebony family: persimmon.

Fungus family: mushroom, yeast, antibiotics.

Ginger family: arrowroot, ginger.

Gooseberry family: gooseberry, currant.

Goose foot (beet) family: beet sugar, cardamom, spinach, chard, kochia, thistle, lamb quarters.

Gourd family: pumpkin, squash, cucumber, cantaloupe, muskmelon, honeydew melon, Persian melon, watermelon, Casaba melon.

Grape family: grape, raisin, cream of tartar, wine, brandy, champagne, wine vinegar.

Heath family: cranberry, huckleberry, blueberry, wintergreen.

Holly family: mate.

Honeysuckle family: elderberry.

Iris family: saffron.

Laurel family: avocado, cinnamon, bay leaves, sassafrass.

Legume family: navy bean, lima bean, kidney bean, string bean, soya bean (oil, flour, lecithin), lentil, black-eyed peas, peanut and oil, jack bean, tonca bean, licorice, gum tragancanth, gum acacia, pinto bean, green pea, field pea, carob (St. John's Bread).

Lily family: asparagus, onion, leek, garlic, sarsaparilla, chives.

Madder family: coffee.

Mallow family: maple syrup, sugar.

May apple family: may apple.

Mint family: peppermint, mint, spearmint, horehound, thyme, marjoram, savory, basil & oregano, sage.

Morning glory family: sweet potato.

Mulberry family: mulberry, fig, hop, breadfruit.

Mustard family: mustard, mustard green, cabbage, cauliflower, broccoli, Brussels sprouts, turnips, rutabagas, kale, collard, kohlrabi, celery cabbage, radish, watercress, colza shoots, Chinese cabbage, kraut, horseradish.

Myrtle family: allspice, cloves, guava.

Nutmeg family: nutmeg, mace.

Oak family: chestnut.

Olive family: green, ripe olive & oil.

Orchid family: vanilla.

Palm family: coconut, date, sago, palm cabbage.

Papaw family: papaw, papaya, papain.

Papaya family: papaya.

Parsley family: parsley, parsnips, carrots, celery, water celery, celeriac, caraway, aniseed, dill, coriander, fennel, celery seed, cummin, angelica.

Pepper family: black pepper, white pepper.

Pine family: juniper, pinion nut.

Pineapple family: pineapple.

Plum family: plum, prune, cherry, peach, apricot, nectarine, wild cherry, almond.

Pomegranate family: pomegranate.

Poppy family: poppy seed.

Potato family: potato, tomato, egg plant, red pepper, cayenne, capsicum, green pepper, chilli, ground cherry, tobacco, belladonna, stramonium, hyoscyamus.

Purslane family: purslane, New Zealand spinach.

Rose family: raspberry, blackberry, loganberry, youngberry, dewberry, strawberry, boysenberry.

Sapodillo family: chicle.

Soapberry family: lichi nut.

Stercula family: cocoa, chocolate, cola bean.

Sponge family: jassava meal, tapioca.

Spurge family: tapioca.

Tea family: tea.

Walnut family: walnut-black, English walnut, hickory nut, pecan, butternut.

Yam family: yam, Chinese potato.

Miscellaneous: honey.

Meat family

Mammals: Beef, veal, milk, butter, cheese, gelatin.

Pork: ham, bacon.

Mutton: lamb.
Horse.
Bear.
Moose.
Rabbit.
Squirrel.
Venison.
Amphibians: Frog.
Reptiles: Turtle, Rattlesnake.
Birds: Chicken, eggs; Goose, eggs; Turkey, eggs; Guinea hen; Pheasant; Duck, eggs; Squab; Grouse.
Fish: Sturgeon (caviar), Salmon, Whitefish, Tuna, Carp, Catfish, Pickerel, Barracuda, Butterfish, Anchovy, Herring, Trout, Chub, Swordfish, Sucker, Bullhead, Muskellunge, Bluefish, Harvestfish, Sardine, Shad, Smelt, Mackerel, Eel, Buffalo, Pike, Mullet, Pompano, Sunfish, Black Bass, Scup, Mealfish, Sole, Codfish, Hake, Perch, Porgy, Drum, Halibut, Squid, Pollack, Snapper, Croaker, Flounder, Rosefish, Haddock, Cusk.
Crustaceans: Crab, Crayfish, Lobster, Shrimp.
Molluscs: Abalone, Mussel, Oyster, Scallop, Clam, Squid.

Food substitution

Foods should not just simply be avoided, something must be put in their place. While it is acceptable for an individual to lose up to half a stone during the initial month of their diet, continued weight loss is both dangerous and worrying. Some of those suffering from food intolerance may already be significantly underweight and so a weight loss of a few pounds may in itself be dangerous. If you are going to embark on a food exclusion diet then you must be sure to substitute the foods you are removing from your diet, both from the point of view of their vitamin and mineral content and with regard to the overall calorie intake.

Most of us are a little overweight, so losing half a stone is often a blessing. Furthermore most people will only need to use fairly simple and straightforward diets, consequently substitution is not much of a problem.

Food reactions

The initial stages of a diet are often a bit stormy. During the first week or two of food avoidance you may well experience food cravings for the foods you have been asked to avoid, this usually indicates a food addiction and is often a sign that the diet will eventually work. Sometimes the symptoms may worsen initially, again this is a good sign and almost invariably means that symptoms will clear after a week or two and you will feel much better.

In order to give the diet an adequate trial, you should persist with your food exclusion rigorously for at least a month. It is often difficult to draw a clear conclusion about the effectiveness of a food exclusion until you have given it a thorough try for between three and five weeks. Sometimes the results will be instantaneous, particularly in children who have behaviour disorders or asthma. In older people, particularly with skin problems such as eczema or arthritic conditions, the diet may take a little longer to have an effect. An initial improvement may occur within the first month, but the full benefit may not be felt for two or three months.

In the initial month, if you stray from your diet, you are quite likely to experience a severe reaction from the foods to which you are intolerant. In time you will become much more food tolerant and the food reactions will usually diminish substantially.

Sticking to the diet

The first month is really a diagnostic period and as a consequence you should stick to the diet as rigorously as you can. If you can avoid the offending foods completely then at the end of this period you will know whether your symptoms are being caused by the offending foods or some other triggers. If you 'cheat' consistently during this first month it will be impossible to draw a clear conclusion, so ultimately the only person you will be cheating on will be yourself! It is inevitable that there will be the odd transgression during this diagnostic period, either because of unavoidable social situations or because of the odd mistake you will make as you get used to the diet. Usually these odd mistakes are not of major importance, but the fewer mistakes you make the clearer the answer will be at the end of the initial period.

General advice about shopping

Most people will have to avoid one or two widely disseminated foods such as milk or wheat. Detailed advice about the major foods, both from the point of view of avoidance and nutritional supplementation, is given in the subsequent sections of this chapter. You will need to be particularly vigilant about the exact food content in prepared and packeted foods. This means that you will need to read the labels on each food packet in some detail so that you know whether the food contains wheat, milk, yeast, etc.

In general it is much safer to buy the individual food constituents and cook all your own foods from basic ingredients so that you know exactly what you are eating. If you are unsure about a prepacked food or the food contents are not clearly labelled, then the safe advice is not to buy or eat that food. If you want to eat muesli for instance, many of the commercially available products contain both milk and wheat. You can however easily make up a very nutritious and tasty breakfast cereal from soya or oat bran with fresh or dried fruit. When you are out of the house it may be difficult to get exactly what you want from a shop, restaurant or snack bar, consequently you should carry some safe foods with you so that you don't feel deprived or become unnecessarily hungry. Raw fruit such as an apple or carrot are often good standbys which fit easily into a handbag or briefcase.

Keeping to your diet means thinking ahead, reading labels and preparing foods from their basic constituents. Once you have got into the habit of doing this it is really very simple and it will allow you to keep to a nutritious diet without feeling deprived or hungry.

What can I cook?

Avoiding foods like potatoes, pork and mushrooms is generally very simple. In the majority of instances these foods are not generally hidden in other foods so you will be able to avoid them by simply not having them. The major foods are however a problem and you may therefore need to develop a repertoire of new recipes depending on which major foods you need to avoid. There are now many recipe books available which involve looking at wheat free, milk free and yeast free cooking. The best books available change from time to time, but a useful selection include:

The Food Watch Alternative Cook Book by Honor J. Campbell (Ashgrove Press, 1986). This is particularly good for wheat and milk free recipes.

The Yeast Connection Cook Book by Dr. W.G. Crook and Hurt Jones (Thorsons, 1988).

Asthma and Eczema by Carol Bennett (Thorsons, 1989). This is particularly useful for milk free diets.

E for Additives by M. Hanson (Thorsons, 1986). This is not a recipe book, but it explains all the E numbers on food packets which you will find particularly useful when trying to do your shopping and organizing a specific food exclusion diet.

These books by no means represent an exhaustive list. There are many other equally good books available from a whole variety of different outlets. If you are having problems with your diet or find it boring, repetitive and unimaginative, then learning some new recipes can be of enormous value. Be adventurous, experiment and try getting some ideas from some of the 'alternative' recipe books that are available.

Who should I see about my diet?

Chapter 6 describes how you can begin to work out your own food sensitivities and develop a food exclusion diet for yourself. Sometimes this can work very simply and straightforwardly with the avoidance of perhaps one major food and a few other associated foods. However, sometimes you can get into deep water; the food avoidance approach may be much more complex than you initially think and furthermore food avoidance alone makes no attempt to look at any of the potential underlying causes for food intolerance. If, therefore, you are going to follow advice from a book or friend about food avoidance, then unless you get a fairly simple, swift and clear-cut result within the first month cease treating yourself. You should then either seek more detailed ecological advice or perhaps look for another approach to resolve your problems.

In our practice the patients who come to see us undergo an initial consultation in which their symptoms and complaints will be discussed in some detail. They may come with the idea that a food exclusion would be an appropriate approach to their problem. While the patient's opinion about which treatment would best suit them is frequently correct, this is not always so and a food exclusion may be a very inappropriate method of management for a particular individual. Sometimes people come just asking us for help and we may recommend a food exclusion as the most appropriate initial treatment. At our first consultation we would then test the patient and work out what foods we would like them to avoid; they will be provided with the appropriate literature to help them with their diet.

We also run a dietary support service through our practice nurses. This allows patients to discuss their diet in some detail with a medically trained individual who is used to dealing with the kind of problems faced by those involved in food exclusion diets. We also offer a 9 to 5 telephone back-up service so that questions and queries can be readily answered rather than waiting for the next consultation. We then review the patient at the end of a month and decide at that point whether the diet has been effective. If the food exclusion has been completely successful, we advise the patient on how best to continue with their diet and when and how they should reintroduce foods. We also offer nutritional advice in order to make sure that their long-term dietary exclusions do not result in vitamin or mineral deficiencies. If our approach has been partially successful or completely unsuccessful we will re-examine our diagnosis and either abandon the diet completely or combine it with other therapeutic techniques.

We appreciate that this approach is based on our own individual experience and has been developed specifically to suit our style of practice. We would not for a moment wish to impose the techniques we use or the clinical approach we have developed on other practitioners. However, there are some important points which we feel those embarking on an ecological approach should consider.

If you have developed an appropriate and effective diet yourself, in order to treat your own problems, you should consult with your family physician to make sure your diet is a sensible one rather than just continuing with it for an indeterminate period of time.

If your initial approaches at sorting your problem out using ecological techniques fail, you should consider consulting a competent practitioner. Unfortunately it is difficult at the present time to define exactly what constitutes a competent practitioner. There are many conventional allergists who have little idea and understanding of clinical ecology. Some are actively disdainful of these techniques in spite of the abundant evidence that attests to their effectivity if used responsibly. The

British Society of Allergy and Environmental Medicine ('Acorns', Romsey Road, Cadnam, Southampton SO4 2NN) is a source of competent medically qualified practitioners working within the field of clinical ecology. Such practitioners use a whole variety of techniques in order to elucidate the appropriate food or chemical intolerance. As with all medical specialties, there are internal differences within this group about the best methods of food testing and ecological management for specific patients or individual diagnoses.

Non-medically trained practitioners offer very variable standards of competence and practice. Some are excellent, with far more knowledge about this area than the vast majority of their conventional colleagues. A number of the non-medically qualified may have basic medical qualifications in nursing or physiotherapy; the current qualifications in osteopathy and chiropractic are also of a very high standard and in many ways directly comparable with the level of competence obtained by a normal medical student.

There are however a number of dubious practitioners of limited competence working within the field of allergy and environmental medicine and at the present time it is impossible to sort out who is competent, capable and responsible from the adverts available in Yellow Pages or your local newspaper. There are no recognized qualifications or nationally competent organisations who are training and registering practitioners within this specific field in the United Kingdom. The real and very unsatisfactory solution for the individual seeking treatment may well be that they have to rely on personal recommendation from friends, family or their doctor if they wish to seek help from someone who is not medically qualified.

Whoever you may wish to see about your problem, if you are going to embark on an ecological approach in order to resolve your symptoms, you will need to be prepared for a minimum of three or four visits over a period of three or four months in order to ascertain whether your problem can be resolved through ecological means. It will take at least this time for an ecologist to be sure that he or she understands your problem and can give you some clear ideas about prognosis and likely response to treatment.

The major foods

In this section we shall define exactly what we mean by the major foods and provide lists of where the major foods are most likely to be found. These lists are not exhaustive but represent a good starting point and a very useful general guide as to what you should avoid if you are on an exclusion diet. We will discuss the major nutritional problems that may be encountered if a particular food is avoided and how these may best be supplemented with either specific vitamin and mineral preparations or foods rich in the nutrients that would be missing from your diet should you avoid a major food. We will also suggest substitutions that can be made when it is necessary to avoid some of the major foods.

Wheat

Foods to avoid:

Wheat flour
Wheatgerm
Wheat-based crispbreads
Wheat biscuits
Wheat breakfast cereals
Wheat-based alcoholic drinks
(whisky, most gins, vodka,
lager and beer)
Wheat bran
Bread

Baking powder
Breadcrumbs
Batter mixes
Cakes and cake mixes
Crumble toppings
Macaroni, spaghetti and
other pasta
Pastry
Pancakes and mixes

You should also check the list of ingredients of the following products:

Baked beans
Chocolate
Coffee (cheap instant) and
drinking chocolate
Cocoa
Cream (imitation)
Chutney, pickles
Custard
Gravy powder/curry powder

Pie fillings
Puddings (instant)
Sausages and patés
Sauces
Stock cubes
Spreads and pastes
Soy sauces
Soups (canned and packet)

Alternatives

Wheat flour: rye flour, brown rice flour, soya flour, potato flour, cornflour, buckwheat flour, arrowroot flour.

Bread: rye bread, oatcakes, pumpernickel bread, rice cakes, rye crispbreads, sprouted grain breads, carrot and raisin breads
Biscuits: flapjacks, macaroons, fruit bars
Cereals: cornflakes, porridge, etc.
Crumble topping/breadcrumbs: oats, sesame seeds, ground rice
Pasta: buckwheat pasta, rice noodles

Wheat flour contains a substantial amount of magnesium and zinc. Wholemeal wheat contains in 100g about 20% of vitamin B-complex and total vitamin E daily requirements. Vitamin B-complex is richest in brewer's yeast or yeast extract, it is also found in brown rice and wheatgerm. Vitamin B12 is found in high concentration in offal such as liver and kidney, but is also present in fatty fish, white fish, eggs and cheese. Vitamin E may be found in soya beans and corn oil. Alternative sources of zinc include liver, brewer's yeast, shellfish, meat and hard cheeses. Alternative sources of magnesium include soya beans, nuts and brewer's yeast.

Wheat is probably one of the most difficult foods to avoid. Intolerance to wheat is frequently associated with intolerance to other grains, particularly oats. However, the vast majority of wheat intolerant individuals will find they are tolerant of some grains such as buckwheat, rye, rice and corn. Some wheat flour substitutes have been suggested, and usually wheat sensitive individuals can find some acceptable grains. Please remember to rotate the grains which you can tolerate otherwise you run the risk of becoming sensitive to other grain products.

Gluten free diets are not the same as wheat free diets. Gluten is contained in the husk of all cereals including wheat. Some gluten free products actually contain wheat.

Milk and milk products
Many people who are milk sensitive are sensitive only to cow's milk and can tolerate sheep's and goat's milk. However some are sensitive to all animal milk and can only use soya milk-based products.

Foods to avoid:

Cow's milk, goat's milk, sheep's milk, condensed, dried, evaporated milk, powdered milk	Butter Cream (fresh) Cheese and dishes cooked with cheese (e.g. quiche)

Whey, lactose, caseinates	Custards
Batter made with milk	Dairy ice cream
Biscuits (some – check contents)	Foods fried in butter
	Malted milk
Cereals (some – check contents)	Sauces (creamed)
	Soups with added milk
Chocolate (milk)	Yoghurt
Cakes in which milk has been used	

Alternatives

Milk: dairy-free coffee creamer, coconut milk (in block form); soya milk, to which apple juice, sugar, and/or calcium may have been added

Butter, margarine: pure sunflower margarine, soya margarines (most – check contents)

Cheese, yoghurt, ice cream: soya cottage cheese, soya hard cheese with herbs, soya yoghurt, tofu or soya ice cream

Milk chocolate: plain chocolate, milk-free carob

Biscuits: animal fat free biscuits

It is vitally important to remember that whey is a milk product. Whey is frequently added to a whole variety of different foods.

Fresh whole cow's milk contains, in 100g, about 120 mg of calcium, 12 mg of magnesium and a small amount of zinc. Milk is also a good source of vitamins D and C, as well as having some vitamin E and B. Vitamin D is found mainly in fish but is also manufactured naturally by sunlight. Vitamin C is obtainable in far higher concentrations from fresh fruit and vegetables. Natural sources of magnesium and zinc have already been mentioned in the section on wheat avoidance. It is really a lack of calcium which is the main problem with milk avoidance. If a young child needs to avoid milk, the baby soya milks are almost always calcium enriched. Some other soya milks are also calcium enriched, but good natural sources of calcium include fish, fortified white flour, root vegetables, nuts, pulses and beans and interestingly enough, sesame seeds. Milk sensitivity is particularly common in young children and prolonged milk avoidance in our opinion requires calcium supplementation. Liquid calcium supplements as well as capsule or pill-based supplements are available.

Milk and milk products are probably among the easiest of the major foods to substitute. There is a whole variety of different soya milks, many of which have slightly different tastes and usually one can be found which is acceptable and palatable. Milk and whey free margarines are now widely available in all the large supermarket chains. Soya-based ice cream and even soya cottage cheese, hard cheeses and yoghurts are now available. If you are able to take goat's and sheep's milk then yoghurt, milk and cheese based on these alternative animal milks should be used with discretion rather than to excess.

Yeast
Yeasts are part of an enormous family of fungi that includes mushrooms, baker's yeast and antibiotics. Some illnesses are caused by fungus, e.g. farmer's lung and candida (thrush). A feature to look for is food which has been around some time, because yeasts need time as well as the right conditions to grow. Many yeasts are invisible to the naked eye. Any products which are fermented, such as wine, will have made use of yeast in their processing. Preserved or dried foods will undoubtedly have yeasts on them, even if they are treated to prevent decay. Some yeasts will be unavoidably taken in as they are everywhere in the air. Clues to the presence of yeast are the descriptions 'malted', 'dried', 'pickled', 'cultured', and 'fermented'. All alcohol contains yeast and must be avoided.

Eating out is not difficult, provided cheese dishes are avoided and any food with vinegar or alcohol as well as pickles and fungi. Bread also has to be avoided, but some plain crispbreads may be acceptable. Salads should not have dressing put on them. Avoid meat with stuffing. Grilled meat without gravy, plain boiled or steamed vegetables, plain grilled fish and omelettes are the safest. Fruit desserts are best avoided and so, of course, is cheese and biscuits.

Foods to avoid

Bread/rolls/croissants	Mushrooms/truffles/other
Pitta bread	fungi
Stuffing made with bread	All cheeses
Yeasted pastries, buns,	Yoghurt
doughnuts	Buttermilk
Summer pudding/fruit	Vinegars – all kinds
charlotte	Ketchups and sauces
Bread and butter pudding	Pickles – all kinds

Chutneys
Sauerkraut
Horseradish
Mint sauce
Malted milk drinks
Malted cereals
Nuts
Monosodium glutomate (Chinese food, flavoured crisps, etc.)
Antibiotics and other drugs derived from mould cultures (pills)
Frozen or canned fruit juices
Citric acid
French mustard
French and other salad dressings

Sweet and sour sauce
Soy sauce
Tomato sauce
Sweet mincemeat
Alcohol – all kinds
Malt
B-complex vitamins
RNA/DNA (pills)
Yeast extract and spreads that contain it
Yeasts of all kinds
Selenium and torula yeasts (supplements)
Dried fruits – all kinds
Fruit skins (orange peel, apple skins, etc.)
Cream of tartar

Alternatives

Bread: soda bread/farls (may contain buttermilk which should be avoided, at least at first), other yeast free breads e.g. manna bread, rye crispbread, crackers (check the ingredients), matzos, oatcakes, rice cakes, some Indian breads (check the ingredients), homemade scones/drop scones; increase intake of pasta, rice, potatoes

Yoghurt: after the first two weeks live yoghurt is acceptable

Salad dressing: lemon, oil, garlic and herbs can be used

Fruit juices: freshly squeezed juices only

Cereals: malt free cereals, porridge oats, homemade muesli, orange crunch

Monosodium glutomate: ask Chinese restaurants/takeaways to leave this out; crisps – either plain or get brands with no additives

Fruit: maximum of three fruits a day, peeled and washed; no fruits may be eaten that cannot be peeled such as berries

Nuts: small amounts of fresh unshelled nuts; avoid peanuts and pistachio nuts

N.B. See also sugar free list.

This diet will reduce the amount of calcium, protein, fibre and fat consumed. Rye crispbreads can be eaten instead of bread, also wholewheat breakfast cereals can be used. Increase the amount of vegetables eaten, especially brassicas. All fruit should be thoroughly washed first, dried and then peeled and eaten immediately. Keep the peel well away from the flesh of the fruit or you may contaminate it with yeast. Make oil/lemon dressings for salads with fresh lemon juice.

The main problem with this diet is the omission of bread, as this could lead to a deficiency of B-complex vitamins. Drop-scones can be made with wholewheat flour. An increase in the amount of liver to 4oz (100g) per week would also help. Natural supplements of B-complex vitamins will probably be made from yeast, in which case synthetic B vitamins would be more suitable if a supplement needs to be taken. Fruit juices should be made from freshly washed and peeled fruit and drunk immediately. If the amount of wholewheat flour used for suitable baking is not increased to at least 1 lb (450g) per week there is a risk of too little cereal fibre in the diet.

Egg

Some people are only allergic to egg white, others to egg yolk, and some are allergic to the whole egg. Grated apple, pectin and methylcellulose, and hemicellulose are sometimes used as binders to replace eggs. You may see albumen in ingredients lists sometimes, which means egg white. E322 indicates the possible inclusion of egg, and foods should be avoided when this E number is listed on the label.

Foods to avoid

Foods made with egg yolk:
Salad cream
Mayonnaise
Hollandaise sauce
Tartare sauce
Marzipan
Mashed potato
Lecithin-enriched margarines, also chocolate, popcorn, packet dessert mixes, bakery products containing lecithin

Foods made with egg white:
Fruit snow
Macaroons
Marshmallows and some sweets
Meringue
Sorbet
Consommé soup
Frosting and royal icing

Foods made with whole egg:

Omelette
Poached egg
Boiled egg
Sponges and cakes
Biscuits
Batter coated foods
Rissoles
Quiches and savoury tarts
Scones made with egg
Muffins
Pasta: macaroni, spaghetti, noodles made with egg
Croissants
Hot cross buns, Bath buns, teacakes, fruit buns
Scrambled eggs
Baked eggs
Pickled eggs
Batter
Desserts
Croquettes
Meat balls, meat loaf
Crumpets
Waffles
Soufflés

Eclairs, choux pastries, profiteroles
Beefburgers, hamburgers
Fish cakes
Welsh cakes
Dropscones
Pancakes
Sauces
Yorkshire pudding
Pastry with egg ('French pastry')
Enriched breads and rolls
Bread and butter pudding
Fried eggs
Scotch eggs
Dried egg
Cookies
Doughnuts
Egg custard
Egg glazed items
Danish pastries
Ice cream
Bedtime drinks
Enriched alcoholic drinks (eggnogs)

One egg contains about one tenth the amount of calcium and one tenth the amount of zinc that is your daily requirement. It also contains a substantial amount of vitamins D and E. Eggs appear to contain chromium as probably the best source of this trace metal, although it can also be obtained from molasses and brewer's yeast.

The nutrients which eggs add to the diet can be replaced by fish, liver and meat. Use thin salad dressings instead of mayonnaise etc. It is possible to make some kinds of cakes without egg at all. When eating out, order very plain food, avoiding batter, soups, sauces and thick dressings as well as desserts, gateaux, ice cream and pastry sweets. Generally speaking, waiters and restaurant staff have no idea of what is actually in the food they serve, so asking the waiter whether there is any egg in a dish is not a very reliable way of finding out.

Some pastas/noodles are made without egg. Look at the

ingredients on the boxes and make a list of the ones which are suitable for this diet as you come across them. Make your own pastry at home and be sure it does not contain egg. Make your own dropscones, without egg, adding more milk to make up the weight. They will be a little rubbery compared with the type made with egg, but are very acceptable. Scones can be made with baking powder and bound with milk or yoghurt.

Some dishes will just have to be avoided, such as soufflés. Use grated apple to bind homemade burgers. Fish can be dipped in milk then flour or cornflour instead of egg batter, before light frying in polyunsaturated oil. On the whole, this is an easy diet to follow and because egg is found in a great number of processed and junk foods it could mean a much healthier one. Eating out is the most difficult part of an egg free diet.

Some supermarkets now sell egg free mayonnaise. Health food shops sell egg substitutes for baking.

Corn or maize

Corn or maize is a common food additive. Many of the added sugar and starch products seen in commercially packaged foods are made from corn, particularly in North America.

Foods to avoid

Corn or maize oil	Cornflour
Cornflakes	Sweetcorn
Ales and beers	Cookies
Aspirin and other tablets	Candies
Baking mixes	Instant coffee
Margarines with corn oil	Custard
Peanut butter	Glucose syrup
Tinned beans and peas	Sandwich spreads
Salad dressings	Quick whips
Sauce mixes	Ice cream
Crisps (some brands)	Popcorn
Instant teas	Stuffings
Tortillas	Sausages
Gravy mixes and cubes	Corn bread
Jams made with glucose	Soy sauce
Imitation cream	Pie fillings
Corn snacks	Chewing gum
Creamed soups	

Many other products are also made from corn, such as adhesives on stamps and envelopes, the lining of paper plates and dishes, talcum powder, toothpaste and even laundry starch. Unless you are particularly corn sensitive it will not be necessary to avoid all these, but you should be aware that corn is probably the most common content of added starch.

Sweetcorn contains a lot of sugar and fibre, important for a healthy diet. The actual nutritional content of cornflour is relatively minimal. It contains small amounts of calcium and magnesium and small amounts of vitamin A, B-complex, D and C. A corn avoidance diet does not require nutritional supplementation, but it will require very careful reading of labels on food packets to make quite sure that you are not having any hidden corn, cornflour or corn sugar. It may well be that if you are particularly corn sensitive, you will simply not be able to have any packaged foods at all, as corn is often added but not mentioned as such on the label.

Soya

Soya is an increasingly used food product and may be found in a wide range of different foods. It must be said that soya sensitivity is not particularly common in Western Europe as we use far less soya-based products than the North Americans. However there are patients who are soya intolerant and the main groups of foods that should be considered as containing soya are:

Bakery goods: occasionally soya bean flour is used as an ingredient of dough mixtures for breads, rolls, cakes and pastries; this keeps them moist and saleable for several days longer

Sauces: soya sauce, Lea & Perrins sauce, Worcester sauce

Salad dressings: many salad dressings and mayonnaise contain soya oil, but only state on the label that they contain vegetable oil

Meats: pork, sausage and luncheon meats may contain soya beans

Sweets: soya flour is used in hard sweets, nut sweets, and caramel; lecithin is invariably derived from soya beans and is used in sweets to prevent drying out and to emulsify the fats

Soya milk

Soya ice cream

Some soups

Fresh soya bean sprouts

Soya bean products, such as textured vegetable protein (T.V.P.)

Soya margarine and butter substitutes

Soya is particularly rich in potassium. Potassium is, however, found in many different foods and fruits, particularly bananas and oranges. It would be difficult in the context of a healthy wholefood diet not to have adequate amounts of potassium. Soya flour also contains almost half the daily requirement of calcium and substantial amounts of magnesium. Methods of substituting calcium and magnesium have already been mentioned in the wheat avoidance list. It is rich in a variety of the vitamins of the B-complex, although if you are able to have yeast, soya avoidance should present no difficulty here. It contains no vitamin C.

In summary, soya is often used as flour, oil, milk substitute and as a replacement for nuts. If you remember this it will be possible to anticipate any inadvertent contact with soya beans and their products.

Sugar

A sugar free diet is very simple, providing you cook all your food from the basic ingredients. Problems begin, however, if you wish to have packaged or instant food. For instance, all jams contain sugar unless it clearly states 'sugar free' on the label. If you wish to buy packaged foods, then read the labels carefully to make sure that no sugar is added. Sugar is added to many items, such as pickles, tomato sauce, many cereals, and a whole host of other items that you may not suspect. Sugar also comes under many guises, such as sucrose, dextrose, fructose, fruit sugars, and honey. If you have any doubt about what the label actually means, then ask. If you cannot get an adequate reply, don't eat the product.

Sugar exclusions are used in two main groups of patients – those with childhood behaviour problems and those with intestinal candida.

Children with behavioural problems may react differently to sugar derived from sugar cane and sugar derived from sugar beet. Consequently raw cane sugar may be acceptable in some instances. Hyperactive children also tend to be fairly safe with fruit sugar (fructose), and many brands of honey, particularly organic honey, as no sugar feeds are given to organically farmed bees.

People with chronic yeast infestation will usually need to avoid all the sugars, fructose, and honey. A basic quality of yeasts is that all of them will ferment on any sugar-based product. As a consequence all the different types of sugars may well trigger yeast growth, although honey and fructose are often less likely to do so than cane and beet sugar.

Please note

● All alcohols are sugar-based, and sugar free diets mean alcohol free diets.

● Sweeteners, unless they specifically state the type of sweetener, should be assumed to be sugar-based. Nutrasweet and saccharin can be used as artificial sweeteners, providing you are not also allergic to these substances. Low calorie or diet drinks usually contain nutrasweet and, unless you react to some other content in diet drinks, they are fine as far as the sugar is concerned.

● Sugar is actually bound into fruit and vegetables (complex food sugars) and they are normally quite safe to eat as the sugar is bound into a complex and usually fibrous chemical structure. As a consequence it is difficult to absorb and so enters the blood stream slowly and in small quantities. Furthermore, usually not enough of it is present at any one site in the digestive system to trigger the growth of yeasts.

● Although in a strict definition of the term sugar is a carbohydrate, added starch or carbohydrate almost always refers to bulking agents, such as corn or wheat flour, and not to sugar.

Foods to avoid

Anything containing cane sugar, beet sugar, molasses, treacle, golden syrup, sucrose, glucose, dextrose, etc.	Squashes
	Alcoholic drinks
	Pickles, chutneys, ketchups, etc.
Sweets	Some packet foods (e.g.
Chocolate	sauces, soups, desserts)
Cakes	Cereals
Biscuits	Some enriched doughs (e.g.
Some tinned food (baked beans, peas, sweetcorn, etc.)	currant teacakes)
	Ice cream, cream substitutes, etc.
Tinned fruit in syrup	
Fizzy drinks	

Alternatives

Sugars: fructose, wild, organic, Mexican or Chinese honey

Sweets: diabetic chocolate, sweets, etc. (occasional treats only)

Drinks: diabetic squash, diet drinks, Aqua Libra, water, unsweetened fruit juice, etc.

Biscuits: some chewy bars, fruit bars, diabetic biscuits, flapjack with honey (occasionally)

Baked beans/tomato ketchup: sugar free varieties
Tinned fruit: varieties in own juice
Cereals, ice cream, jam, nut butter: sugar free varieties (check
  contents)

Citrus fruits
The avoidance of citrus fruits often means the avoidance of
citric acid as well. It is largely a question of reading labels and a
general guideline for citrus fruit avoidance is given below.
Citrus fruits include orange, lemon, grapefruit, lime, tangerine, satsuma, clementine, ugli, angostura.

The whole fruit or just the juice, the skin or the flavour are
used in manufacturing:

Sweets and confectionery	Pickles
Ice cream	Chutneys
Flavourings	Lemon tea
Candied peel	Oil/lemon salad dressing
Fruit squashes and drinks	Fish and poultry dishes
Fruit juice – canned, frozen	Marinade for kebabs
or in cartons	Sweet and sour sauce
Cakes, biscuits, cookies	Orange flower water
Cheesecake	Lemonade
Sponge	Lemon barley water
Jellies	Bioflavonoid supplements un-
Flavoured yoghurts	less synthetic
Angostura bitters	Citrus flavoured toothpaste
Sauces	

Some E numbers indicate the inclusion of citrus, and food
should be avoided where these E numbers are listed on the
label: E330, E331, E332, E333, E334, E440(A), E450(B),
E472(C).
The major risk with avoiding citrus is that your diet may be low
in vitamin C. Vitamin C can be obtained from almost any fresh
fruit and vegetables. If you intend to obtain the vitamin C
largely from vegetables, then eat them raw or very lightly
cooked. The recommended daily vitamin C intake is only 50
mg; if you wish to supplement it is easy to do so as its available
in almost every pharmacy and health food shop. Remember to
take a citric acid free supplement. In general, however, supplementation should not be necessary if you eat fresh vegetables
once a day.

Specific diseases associated with allergy

Salicylates

Salicylates are not a food in themselves, but are common natural chemicals found in many different foods. They have been implicated as a very important factor in childhood food intolerance, particularly in hyperactive children. The concept of natural food chemicals running through whole ranges of different foods, and triggering food sensitivity has been discussed in some detail in Chapter 9. The list below provides the best information we have about salicylate content in common foods. There are, however, authorities who would argue with this salicylate list, so the situation is far from clear.

High levels

Dried fruit	All berries and	Cherries
Oranges	currants (e.g.	Apricots
Grapes	redcurrants)	Plums
Apples (except	Courgettes	Avocado
Golden Delicious)	Pineapples	Melons
Aubergine	Grapefruit	Licorice
Lychees	Peaches	Watercress
Strong mints	Nectarines	Asparagus
Cucumber	Tomatoes and	Peppers
Tinned sweetcorn	tomato products	Water chestnuts
All spices and spice	Broad beans	Coffee
sauces	Radishes	Tea
Peanuts	Almonds	

Moderate levels

Pears	Golden Delicious	Lemons
Rhubarb	apples	Passion fruit
Pomegranates	Mango	Broccoli
Sweet potato	Paw-paw	Mushrooms
Carrots	Parsnips	Marrow
Spinach	Beetroot	Cauliflower
Fresh sweetcorn	Onion	Garlic
Pistachio nut	Potato (with peel)	Brazil nut
Coconut	Walnut	Hazelnut

Low or nil levels

Pears (peeled)	Potato (peeled)	Lettuce
Celery	Cabbage	Bamboo shoots

Swede	Dried beans and	Lentils
Green beans	peas	Leeks
Shallots	Sprouts	Cashew nut
Herb tea	Parsley	Malted milk drinks
	Dandelion coffee	

Note: Other foods, except those containing or derived from corn, have negligible amounts of salicylate.

In general, avoiding the high and moderate levels of salicylates is usually enough, although in particularly sensitive individuals, all three groups need to be avoided. The major problem is finding fruit and vegetables that can be eaten with impunity, and also drinks – especially for children also on a milk free diet. This may necessitate some experimental recipes! A salicylate free diet does mean the diet may be low in vitamin C, but in general it will be adequate for most of the other essential vitamins and minerals. Supplementation with artificially made vitamin C would be useful if people on a salicylate free diet cannot find any vegetables to their taste.

Conclusion

In this chapter we have tried to provide you with some commonsense advice about organizing your diet. When starting a diet it is essential to plan and think carefully about the foods you can and can't have. Rotate your foods and substitute rather than simply take foods out, so that you make sure that you have a nutritionally adequate diet. We have tried where possible to give alternative food suggestions, as well as pointing out some nutritional pitfalls that can occur with the avoidance of major foods. If you use your common sense, read the labels and are prepared to be adventurous with your cooking, a food avoidance diet can often be fun as well as therapeutically effective.

CHAPTER 21

Where do we go from here?

This book has suggested a number of controversial ideas, and they contain the seeds for the next steps forward. Before these steps can be taken effectively, a lot of groundwork remains to be done.

Increased recognition of environmentally caused illness

The existence of environmentally caused illness needs to be more widely recognized by doctors and patients alike. It is still a minority approach to illness by doctors and by many it is regarded as cranky. Convincing evidence is steadily accumulating that many patients are ill because of their environment. There is little evidence, however, that the publication of learned papers influences the way doctors practise. Changing medical fashion is probably the biggest factor in affecting the way medicine is practised, much to the continued embarrassment of the bastions of academic medicine. Hopefully this book will be a step in the right direction as we have tried to be critical of both the conventional and environmentally-based approach and therefore we feel we have presented a balanced view.

Education of doctors

Doctors receive no training in the management of ecological illness. Those that have an interest have usually picked up their expertise from patients, and through various books often written for the lay public. A few have attended one of the rare training courses in environmental medicine, more widely available in America than in the UK. Many doctors with such an interest often suffer from environmentally-based illness themselves. Our experience has been that there was nowhere for us to go to learn ecology, when our interest began in this area, hardly a good basis for us to develop our skills. This situation has been remedied to a limited extent, and more courses and books are now available. One day medical students may learn this approach as undergraduates, but this is probably many years away.

Research

As must be apparent from this book, ecology is full of unexplained findings, indicating an obvious need for more research. In terms of research funding, ecology has been a Cinderella but there are signs that things may be changing. Research is needed on two fronts, clinical trials and basic mechanisms. The major lack is research into basic mechanisms of sensitivity, as it is only when we understand these better that we can usefully modify treatment programmes. More innovative work is needed, as conventional explanations of allergy break down when applied to ecology.

Holism

Holism seems to be the up and coming fashion, and has come to us in the recognition and treatment of all aspects of the patient's problem. We believe that this is a major step forward, as it encourages a broad view of illness and discourages a narrow specialist approach. The specialist approach still dominates, but things are changing. Ecologists themselves have often been guilty of a narrow approach, and they will have to stand back and recognize the existence of underlying causes in environmentally-based illness. Only when a holistic approach, as exemplified in general practice, carries the same sort of respect given to specialist medicine, can these new approaches be researched in an unprejudiced manner.

Changes in the patient's environment

So far all the steps forward have largely been directed at doctors; but what about the patient? People are now more environmentally aware, as it becomes generally accepted that we live on a planet with finite resources. Green political movements are gaining ground everywhere in the civilized world, so much so that the major parties are now adopting important environmental initiatives within their programmes. Pollution is universally recognized and encouraging steps are being taken to improve our environment and to lessen pollution. These ideas will begin to find political expression as green politics becomes more powerful. It is likely that these innovative political movements will become of major importance over the next half century.

On a personal level, everyone would be wise to limit ecologically dangerous exposure. The use of aerosol sprays, garden pesticides and weedkillers and artificial fertilizers should be stopped. The wise person will grow the majority of his or her own food requirements, without chemical help. Drug exposure should be kept to a minimum and processed foods of all sorts should be avoided where possible. All these measures will lead to a more healthy life.

Governmental action to control car use

There can be no doubt that a major cause of urban pollution, and indeed the greenhouse effect, is the ordinary motor car which the majority of us drive every day. If we are going to preserve our planet, and reduce the incidence of allergic disease, there can be no doubt that control of car use is a major task we are all going to have to face. This issue has been consistently fudged by practically every government worldwide so far. Time is running out. We need to concentrate on efforts to make the car safe, such as by making catalytic converters on exhausts compulsory, to name but one measure. We need to put a great deal of thought and funds into finding other ways to make the car safe, or looking at other ways of transportation which do not involve the burning of fossil fuels. Any legislation to simply stop people driving cars simply would not work, as in all modern societies transportation by car is an integral part, and very few of us indeed would part with our cars on the basis that doing that would lead to a cleaner world. This solution simply would not work. We see therefore the taming of the motor car as being a major task for international and local government over the next few years, as a major means of controlling the increased incidence of allergic disease.

Multinational and governmental action

Perhaps the most important changes have to be brought about by multinational companies and governments. Ironically, multinationals often appear to wield more power than governments, but so long as their decisions are based purely on economic considerations, we can't hope to move much further forward. Environmental awareness doesn't make profits, but it enables us all to live a more healthy and fulfilled life. There are signs that multinationals will respond to public pressure, but much still remains to be done.

Governments will hopefully continue to pass anti-pollution legislation, such as encouraging people to use lead free petrol by making it cheaper to buy. As a result of public campaigning, it now appears at least possible that lead will be banned from petrol in the UK within the foreseeable future. Many other well directed, vigorous and hard-hitting public campaigns are needed, as this is how change is brought about – the anti-nuclear campaign is a good example. Organized campaigns against agrochemicals are becoming more widespread and coherent, and may ultimately lead to more effective action in this area. We hope that this book will encourage the many people who are trying to change things, but appear to be losing all the time, that success will come if only they persist.

In conclusion, we have tried to present a balanced view of environmentally caused illness, indicating areas where it ought to change. We have also given as much advice as has been possible in a book of this size for use by the man or woman in the street. We haven't made it a book of diets or of food lists, even though these are included. We have tried to make people think and so we have been deliberately controversial – it seemed a waste of effort to write the same book on environmental medicine that other people have written. The next few years will show us whether we have been successful or not.